The 7 Mindsets

To Live Your Ultimate Life

The 7 Mindsets
To Live Your Ultimate Life

An Unexpected Blueprint
for an Extraordinary Life

Scott Shickler
&
Jeff Waller

Creators of the 7 Mindsets

For every book purchased, a book will be donated to a student through the Magic Wand Foundation, a non-profit organization dedicated to empowering youth to live their dreams.

The 7 Mindsets To Live Your Ultimate Life
An Unexpected Blueprint for an Extraordinary Life

Copyright © 2011 by Scott Shickler and Jeff Waller
Revised Edition, Published 2017

Author photographs by Haigwood Studios Photography

Copyeditor: Jadd Shickler
Contributing Editor: Vincent Begley
Cover Design & Layout: Annisa Olson Jones
Composition: Alice M. Ormiston

ISBN: 978-1-68102-575-9

Printed in the United States of America

"A candle loses nothing by lighting another candle."

—Father James Keller

We dedicate this book to our children

Jaxson, Hayden, Daniel, Ana Lucia and Sienna.
You make the world a brighter place.

It is also dedicated with love to

Grace and Lilly,
our blueprints for extraordinary wives.

What people are saying about
The 7 Mindsets to Live Your Ultimate Life:

"The *7 Mindsets* book is fascinating and spot-on. It's a new classic in the company of *Think and Grow Rich* and *How to Win Friends and Influence People*."

Larry Hart
Group Chair at Vistage International, GA

"Throughout my career, I have had the opportunity to meet many successful people, and you can immediately tell they have determined mindsets that drive them nonstop towards their goals. Every parent and teacher should be sharing the 7 *Mindsets* with our children for them to flourish in this new, highly competitive global marketplace."

Famous Dave Anderson
Founder, World's Best BBQ and America's Best-Tasting Ribs!

"Shickler and Waller have hit the bullseye. The *7 Mindsets* are exactly what's needed to transform an ordinary life into an extraordinary one."

Dahlynn McKowen
Coauthor, *Chicken Soup for the Soul*

"It is so powerful to observe the impact of the *7 Mindsets* on students. It's like the veil that is covering the secret to success is lifted and they begin to realize that it is within their control to embrace the mindsets that will ultimately change the trajectory of their lives."

Amy Hodgson
Educator /Superintendent in Michigan

"The *7 Mindsets* offers one of the most phenomenal and revolutionary messages of our time. The theories have inspired a great upgrade in my thinking towards living an extraordinary life, and it is spreading very quickly among young people here in Africa, poised to bring about a much needed generational shift."

Adeniyi Bankole
Lawyer/Social Entrepreneur, Nigeria

"The *7 Mindsets* have been an important turning point in my life. Not only did I start thinking like a global citizen, but I have developed a passion to make the world a better place. I am now using them as a daily compass for my life, and highly recommend others do the same."

James Mwakichako
Student, Kenya

"I have seen firsthand how the *7 Mindsets* have transformed students from around the world. Students are equipped with principles that help them take ownership of their lives, focus their time and energy, and positively impact the world around them. The world would be a better place if all students were taught the *7 Mindsets!*"

Bill Schulte
Educator, FL

"The *7 Mindsets* have proved to me that I can live my dreams; that they become very realistic once you define them and start taking the necessary steps. I believe their greatest power is in inspiring young people from all over the world to live better lives and work together to build a better society and planet!"

Itzel Polin
Student, Mexico City, Mexico

"No one is better suited to understand the trends and issues of today's teenagers than themselves. The research and message of the *7 Mindsets* not only empower teenagers to take ownership of the challenges facing their generation, but also give them tools to help them immediately take action. I have personally seen the insights of the *7 Mindsets* put into action, and it is nothing short of awesome."

Wesley Bender
Youth Leader, YMCA, GA

"Working with business professionals, I hear comments about the apathy of teens today. Through the mindsets, young adults are given a vehicle to put their energy and imagination to work. The results are absolutely incredible, and may be exactly what we need to change the business community and the world."

April Farlow
Leadership Instructor/Consultant

"The *7 Mindsets* were planted in my son's heart at the right time and have influenced him to pursue extraordinary achievements. From starting his own business when he was thirteen to his current leadership positions at school to pursuing his dreams in nuclear engineering, it all started by living the mindsets."

Manual Carvallo
Parent

"If you want to transform your business, then every employee should read this book. The *7 Mindsets* will raise the level of performance for everyone who puts them into action."

Susan Wilson Solovic
NY Times Best Selling Author & CEO, *It's Your Biz*

TABLE OF CONTENTS

The 7 Mindsets

To Live Your Ultimate Life

A Message from the Authors

The first edition of this book was published after our initial investment of several years studying thousands of the world's happiest and most successful people.

Our simple conclusion was that happy and successful people think differently—they have certain mindsets in common that allow them to experience more joy, gratitude, and connectedness than others.

Through this revelation, we identified the 7 Mindsets at the heart of lives filled with passion, purpose and the drive to succeed, and detailed them in the book you're about to read.

The response was overwhelmingly positive. Tens of thousands of books were purchased, read, downloaded, listened to and shared with friends, family and colleagues around the world.

We were invited to give hundreds of presentations to help others better understand the 7 Mindsets and learn to incorporate them into their personal and professional lives.

What happened next was life-changing. A movement began. We call it the Mindset Revolution.

We decided to apply our findings in schools to see if we could teach students the 7 Mindsets and, more importantly, whether this could positively impact their social and academic development.

The short answers were that we could and it did.

As of this writing, we are now working with hundreds of thousands of students from kindergarten through high school to learn the 7 Mindsets each week.

The results have been nothing short of amazing, from a documented positive impact on academic performance and student behavior to sustained increases in both Grit and Resilience.

We now have training programs across the country to teach educators how to bring the 7 Mindsets to their schools and online programs for parents to bring the mindsets into their homes.

Our next goal? To reach and support students by the millions.

We hope you'll find this book empowering on a personal level and, if so moved, that you'll join us in helping bring these valuable lessons to every student in every corner of the world.

With gratitude!

Scott Shickler

&

Jeff Waller

Introduction

I don't know how many people in the world can look back and recognize the moment that changed their lives, but I'm lucky enough to be able to do so.

My life changed on the day I walked into a Boys & Girls Club in Newark, New Jersey.

It all started when I was asked to be a guest speaker one Saturday afternoon to a group of students. I had never been to Newark and was actually a bit afraid. At that time, Newark was considered one of the most dangerous cities in the country. It was not only number one in auto theft, but also the leader in the latest craze of carjacking.

So there I was, talking to a group of ten year olds about the only thing I felt confident speaking about: business. I wasn't a teacher. I was an entrepreneur fresh out of college. I wasn't even sure if ten year olds could comprehend the concept of business, let alone be interested in how businesses worked. Unsure of what to expect, I was introduced as a business owner, and my heart warmed when I saw a spark of interest in their eyes. Out of curiosity, I asked if any of them were interested in starting their own companies one day, or maybe even being their own bosses. Almost every hand went up, and I'm sure I had a startled look on my face. Then a student asked how he could become a business owner like me, and sort of leaned toward me in anticipation. I wasn't expecting this question, and, as I paused for a moment to try to respond in a way that made sense to a ten year old, the teacher standing in the back of the room chimed in.

The teacher told the students that, in order to start their own business, they needed to graduate from high school, go to college, get an MBA, write a business plan, and raise a lot of money. When they had done all that, they would have a three out of ten chance of success in a business of their own. In less than thirty seconds, that teacher had completely changed the energy in the room. I watched as the students lost their enthusiasm and many literally slumped down in their chairs.

The strange thing was, I had heard this advice before … when I was a kid filled with curiosity. But having lived a different experience than the one the teacher was describing, I knew things not only could be different, but *should* be different. I told the kids that their teacher had indeed pointed out *one* way to become business owners, but that I knew of another way for all of them to become their own bosses much sooner—perhaps even in a matter of days or weeks. With that simple statement of hope, they all perked up again.

Over the next four weeks, I continued to volunteer. I took the students to a local wholesaler, giving them each ten dollars in seed capital so they could buy merchandise to start their business. I showed them how to make posters, flyers, and marketing materials. I encouraged them to come up with names for their businesses, give themselves titles, and I had business cards made up for each of them. We set up a market in the lobby of the Boys & Girls Club where the fledgling entrepreneurs sold their wares. Afterwards, I took them to a local bank and helped them open savings accounts to hold their newly earned money. Everything appeared to be going great, and they seemed to be natural entrepreneurs … until I got a call telling me the club director wanted to talk to me before I taught another class.

With some trepidation, I entered her office.

The Director said to me, "Mr. Shickler," then paused, which didn't sound like a good start to me. "I've been getting a lot of calls from parents about this new program we're offering and, interestingly, I didn't even know we had a new program."

I immediately said that it wasn't really a program—that I was just trying to teach the students about business.

That's when she pointed to a boy playing outside her office and asked, "Do you see that kid over there? Last month he stole a car. The month before that, he stole two cars!"

I said, "You're kidding, right? Jamal?" Jamal was one of the students in my business class. "He stole a car? He's only ten years old. He can't even see over the steering wheel!" Flustered and not sure what to do, and almost fearing the answer to my question, I asked, "What has he done this month?"

"That's just it!" she replied. "He hasn't done anything wrong all month! He seems really engaged in your program."

I was still a little unsure where things were headed. "Actually," I timidly interjected, "I don't really have a program."

The director smiled and said, "You do now."

My life changed that day, and little did I know that I would spend the next two decades teaching entrepreneurship, financial literacy, and personal achievement to tens of thousands of students and educators across the country and around the world. I've written books, started multi-million-dollar education companies, and seen my work featured in an array of media from CNN, ABC and NBC News to *The Wall Street Journal* and *The New York Times*.

This book, however, is by far the most important piece of work I, together with my colleague and co-author, Jeff Waller, have ever done. It is the culmination of years of research and millions of dollars invested in search of the answer to a simple question: "If every kid wants to grow up to live a happy and successful life, why do so few achieve it?"

Every parent wants his or her child to grow up to be happy and successful. Every teacher wants the same for his or her students. Billions of dollars are spent each year on public and private schools, and by a myriad of non-profit organizations on one seemingly simple goal...preparing young people for successful lives. Unfortunately, however, for all the billions of dollars and hours spent, things are just not working.

One doesn't have to look far to find the signs of failure. One out of three students who enter first grade will not graduate from high school. One in five children will experience depression before they become adults. Each day in America, fifty young people try to take their own lives. In 2010, there were as many bankruptcies as there were newly minted college graduates. Whatever one's measure of success and happiness, these young people surely don't have it.

However, do not think these are simply the typical challenges of navigating through adolescence that adulthood will change. A 2010

Introduction

Gallup Poll found that only twenty percent of adults are passionate about what they do for a living, leaving eighty percent wishing they were doing something else. It seems that the new status quo is living a life of unrealized dreams. Does it have to be this way? Not according to our research.

We all know people who seem to live lives of great happiness and joy. They've discovered peace and a real sense of meaning in their lives. Their success stands out from the crowd, and while they make up a small percentage of society, there is no reason it has to remain this way. Happy and successful people have always existed, and we believe that happiness and success are within reach for all of us.

What you are about to discover in this book are the results of our revolutionary research and its breakthrough conclusions. We studied some of the happiest and most successful people of all time. We looked at what drove them and what conditions existed that propelled them and allowed them to achieve their Ultimate Lives. Eventually, we saw a definite pattern emerge and were able to identify the individual pieces that produced the pattern of success. It is that pattern that's at the core of this book, what we call *The 7 Mindsets*.

In this book, Jeff and I will share the results of our research, some of which will astound you, and all of which holds the key to helping you achieve your own level of greatness. We hope our discovery will empower and inspire you to live your Ultimate Life. I must warn you, however, that Jeff and I have a hidden agenda. We believe that many of the world's challenges are going to be solved only in the hearts and minds of young people. If we had magic wands, we would empower all youth around the world to live their Ultimate Lives and bring positive change to their communities. Perhaps our magic wand is the content of this book. We believe we can help create a generational shift, one in which young people live to their greatest potential and seek exciting, creative, and meaningful ways to make a positive impact on the world.

Today, I feel like I am much more than just a businessman. When I think back on the nervous, uncertain young man walking into that Newark Boys & Girls Club, I can't help but smile and shake my head. I didn't know exactly what I was going to do for the next two hours, let alone the next two decades. All I knew was that I wanted to help some young people find success. I did that then, and I am still doing it today. It's been a long journey, but it's been a great one; and it has led me to believe that I can empower millions of people to live their Ultimate Lives.

The 7 Mindsets have the power to unlock the door to success and happiness. Jeff and I invite you to explore the unexpected blueprint for an extraordinary life. Empowered by the 7 Mindsets, everything is indeed possible.

Scott J. Shickler
Roswell, GA

The Great Paradox
Chapter 1

"We cannot solve the problems we face with the same level of thinking that created them."

—Albert Einstein

The Burning Question

If everyone wants to grow up to live a happy and successful life, why do so few achieve it?

This simple question launched a multi-year, multi-million-dollar research project. In the first phase of our research, we studied happy and successful people throughout history, hoping to identify important similarities. The second phase of our research uncovered why the majority of people fall short of reaching their desired level of happiness and success. In the third and final phase of our research, we developed a methodology to teach our findings to young people in a meaningful and sustainable way.

The research is groundbreaking, and the results are both surprising and revolutionary. This book contains our findings, as well as a blueprint for living a life of greater potential, meaning and significance. An Ultimate Life is one filled with passion, happiness, and extraordinary success. We will attempt to be as clear and straightforward as possible in demystifying what we learned.

"If you want to know how to get where you want to go, listen to the people coming back from where you want to be."

—Anonymous

History Holds the Answers

The self-help industry generates *billion* of dollars a year. There is no shortage of books, CDs, DVDs, and seminars on how to live a better life. Research shows that the majority of typical self-help customers were previous purchasers of self-help material. This is one reason why self-help has been referred to as "shelf-help"—customers don't seem to find solutions that work for them, so they hop from one product to the next, filling their bookshelves along the way.

Many self-help gurus believe that most people are simply hungry and eager to learn more strategies and wouldn't buy self-help products if they didn't work. But in spite of all the self-help strategies being pitched, more and more people seem to be miserable and falling short of their desired goals.

It doesn't help that there is conflicting advice on the subject of personal achievement. It's like finding a needle in a haystack. Where do you begin? What books should you read? The comedian George Carlin once said in a stand-up routine, "I went to a bookstore and asked the saleswoman, 'Where's the self-help section?' She said if she told me, it would defeat the purpose."

Finding the right advice is only part of the challenge. Making the necessary change is what derails most people. So we decided to begin our research studying those who've managed to find the right advice and implement changes in their lives. We have nicknamed this group the *ultra successful* because they do stand out from the crowd. It was important to research people throughout time, from the famous to the relatively unknown, from all walks of life and regions of the world. You will recognize the names of many people in our research, but we also studied hundreds of seemingly ordinary people who found a way to live lives filled with greater joy and personal achievement than most.

Happiness and success are subjective concepts, but we measured our results according to the norms of the day. We all know people who have money but are miserable. We also know people who seem to have few material luxuries, yet they radiate joy and zest for life. All of these factors were considered as we looked to see if we could find significant similarities. This is not a book that outlines get-rich-quick strategies, or focuses solely on the wealthy and famous. While many of the people we studied had accumulated more money in their lives than they ever imagined possible, others showed no real interest in generating wealth and possessed their own unique measures for success. We were in search of people who had found ways to live lives filled with passion, meaning, and a strong sense of purpose and achievement. What follows is an overview of our research process.

We Studied the Studies

Throughout history, great minds and organizations have analyzed and studied happiness, achievement, and success. We started our research by examining the large body of existing research. We studied the writings of the ancient Chinese masters including Lao Tzu and Confucius. We studied the works and lives of the Greek philosophers including Aristotle, Plato, and Socrates. We analyzed the works of the Roman Stoic philosophers, including Epictetus and Marcus Aurelius. We reviewed the lives and works of the Middle Eastern philosophers such as Rumi, and the European thinkers including Voltaire, Descartes, and Da Vinci. We studied the influential works of the twentieth century Industrial Revolution including those of Napoleon Hill, Dale Carnegie, and W. Clement Stone. Lastly, we analyzed the fifty-million-dollar research project on global happiness and other research conducted by Dr. Martin Seligman, Director of the Positive Psychology Center at the University of Pennsylvania.

We Read the Landmark Books

With millions of books available through Amazon, we needed to be selective in our source material. We elected to focus on bestselling titles that have appeared to stand the test of time and critical review. A complete list can be found in the resource section at the back of this book. A sample of the books used in our research includes:

Think and Grow Rich by Napoleon Hill
The 7 Habits of Highly Effective People by Stephen Covey
Man's Search for Meaning by Viktor Frankl
Authentic Happiness by Martin Seligman
The Success Principles by Jack Canfield
The 7 Spiritual Laws of Success by Deepak Chopra
Now Discover Your Strengths by Marcus Buckingham
Good to Great by Jim Collins
Happy for No Reason by Marci Shimoff
The Passion Test by Janet & Chris Attwood
The Alchemist by Paulo Coelho
The Purpose Driven Life by Rick Warren
The Secret by Rhonda Byrne
The Power of Positive Thinking by Dr. Norman Vincent Peale
The Art of Happiness by the Dalai Lama
The Four Agreements by Don Miguel Ruiz
The Power of Now by Eckhart Tolle

Unlimited Power by Anthony Robbins
Maximum Achievement by Brian Tracy
Excuses Begone by Dr. Wayne Dyer

We Analyzed the Ultra Successful

Since the time of the Renaissance, thousands of extraordinary lives have been documented. We felt it critical that these lives be analyzed to find significant similarities. We researched great artistic minds like Da Vinci, Michelangelo, and Shakespeare. We reviewed the philosophies of some of history's foremost scientific thinkers, including Isaac Newton, Charles Darwin, and Albert Einstein. We examined the iconic American success stories of John Rockefeller, Henry Ford, Thomas Edison, Andrew Carnegie, Cornelius Vanderbilt, J.P. Morgan, and others. We studied the lives of brave social change agents like Gandhi, Mother Teresa, and Martin Luther King, Jr. We analyzed accounts of epic political leaders including Nelson Mandela, Winston Churchill, and Abraham Lincoln. We read the autobiographies and biographies of daring entrepreneurs like Sir Richard Branson, Bill Gates, and Anita Roddick. We considered celebrated athletes including Michael Jordan, Wilma Rudolph, and Pelé, and the lives of such extraordinary artists and entertainers as Oprah Winfrey, Will Smith, Shakira, and others like them.

We Conducted Live Interviews

Getting to the heart of the matter included interviewing over 400 successful individuals and authors who focus on happiness, achievement, and success. Some of the people interviewed included billionaire Richard Branson; Wally "Famous" Amos; Brian Tracy; Les Brown; Jack Canfield & Mark Victor Hanson, co-authors of the bestselling *Chicken Soup for the Soul* series; Ben & Jerry;

Fred DeLuca, founder of Subway; Earl Graves, founder of *Black Enterprise* magazine; Steve Forbes, Editor of *Forbes* magazine; Snowden McFall, author of *Fired Up!;* Dr. Wayne Dyer; Robert Kiyosaki, author of *Rich Dad Poor Dad*; Dr. Dennis Waitley, author of *The Psychology of Winning*; Steve Jobs; Dr. Ken Blanchard, global leadership expert; Cheryl Richardson, co-author of *You Can Create an Exceptional Life;* and Anita Roddick, founder of The Body Shop.

We Researched With Our Students

Our education company has served millions of educators and youth around the world. We have developed knowledge through firsthand experience on the thought patterns, perspectives, and expectations of teens. We understand how youth view happiness and success. We are intimately familiar with the common advice delivered by parents and educators on how to be successful. We understand what motivates students and, of equal importance, the things that demotivate them. It is this youth empowerment expertise that ultimately allowed us to translate our findings into a language and structure both relevant and engaging for teens and adults. Through the years, we have learned to translate sophisticated content into a usable and sustainable form.

The Revolutionary Results

After thousands of hours of research, in excess of 400 interviews, a comprehensive analysis of comparative data from other research projects, and the deconstruction of over 100 books, our results were astounding.

We'll begin by telling you what the happiest and most successful

14

people don't have in common. It's not their genders, ethnicities, or where they live in the world. It has nothing to do with whether they came from loving homes or broken ones. It doesn't matter if their families come from money, are middle class, or impoverished. It's not even connected to how far they advanced in school or the skill sets they acquired along the way. While all of these things seem important, they proved to be only surface attributes. We found resounding evidence that patterns of happiness and success come from both genders and all ethnicities; from the well-educated and the unschooled; from those with means to those without; and from those with loving parents to those who were adopted, abandoned, and even abused.

Equally important is that people who do not view themselves as happy and successful also come from both genders, all ethnicities, loving and dysfunctional homes, households with Ivy League parents as well as parents who were high school dropouts, professional and blue collar homes, and across the wide economic spectrum of the haves and have-nots. The game-changing patterns of happiness and success are not based on one's personal history, nor on the common belief that "it's not what you know, but who you know."

Our findings alone can save you a lifetime of heartache. We hope your brain is spinning as our research results challenge much of what's thought of as "conventional wisdom."

What Do the Ultra Successful Have in Common?

Simply put, it's the way they think. The happiest and most successful people we researched have certain mindsets in common. Specifically, we identified seven common mindsets. While it was not essential that every research subject possess all seven mindsets at all times, we did find that the ultra successful, the happiest and the most accomplished people in the study, actively embraced the majority of the mindsets at different points in their lives. We have labeled these commonalities *The 7 Mindsets to Live Your Ultimate Life,* and there is a chapter in this book devoted to each of them.

The Great Paradox

As expected, our research revealed many of the usual predictors of success and happiness in life. What we did not expect was that, upon finding a series of mindsets common to those we call the ultra successful, we also learned that not only are the vast majority of people not living those mindsets, but most are thinking and acting in direct contradiction to them. Evidence suggests that a majority of society is applying what we have labeled *the counter mindsets.* To compound the matter, most teachers and parents actually *teach* the counter mindsets, because that's what they have been taught will lead to the good life. Unfortunately, for most people, the counter mindsets have become the status quo and eventually drive individuals to live lives of moderate success and fleeting happiness, at best.

In the next chapter, we will address the counter mindsets and set the stage for a transformational mind shift … one with the potential to empower you to live your Ultimate Life.

Change Your Mindsets, Change Your Life
Chapter 2

"Our environment, the world in which we live and work, is a mirror of our attitudes and expectations."

–Earl Nightingale

In the first decade of the 21st century, it was estimated that more than a billion children were deprived of food, and more than twenty percent of them were chronically malnourished. Twice as many people died in the 20th century from war-related violence than in the 19th century. Most experts now predict these numbers to double again by the end of the 21st century. The global economy is in turmoil, and many believe we are systematically destroying our planet. In the United States, dropout rates are increasing, depression is growing, and violence and drug abuse continue to be prevalent. At a time when we have more than we've ever had, we seem more at odds than ever with living lives of true happiness and meaning. Worse, we seem to have catastrophic issues with very few answers. If the 7 Mindsets have been around throughout recorded history, why do so many people not fully understand them? And perhaps even more perplexing, why have the majority of people adopted the exact opposite mindsets? This chapter will explain some possible theories and provide the foundation for a positive mind shift.

Let's Go to the Flea Circus

Now a thing of the past, flea circuses started in England around 1830. They grew in popularity among circuses and carnivals around the world for a hundred years, then ultimately disappeared from the entertainment landscape by the end of the 1960s. During the height of their popularity, there were not only people who willingly paid money to watch fleas perform circus acts, but also those who even became professional flea trainers ... and it's the flea trainers who help shed some light on the societal issues of our time.

The process of training fleas was quite simple. Dozens of fleas were gathered and placed in a glass jar with a lid. Fleas are known for their ability to jump, but as they naturally jumped inside the jar, they would bang their heads on the lid. After just two days of this "training," they began to adjust the height of their jumps so they would avoid banging into the lid. The trainer could then remove the lid of the jar, and the fleas would maintain their same jumping height. Even though they could easily clear the confines of the jar, they would no longer jump high enough to escape.

What's even more interesting is that, when the fleas reproduced, they taught their offspring to jump only as high as the imaginary lid. One can only suppose that the parent fleas had the best interests of their babies at heart. After all, who wants their young to experience pain? Little did they know that they were limiting the future potential of several generations of fleas.

Virus of the Mind

Every day, a virus wakes up with a simple list of things to do: infiltrate a host, spread throughout the host, infect another host, and repeat … all day, every day. There are biological viruses that are transmitted through human contact. There are computer viruses that carry programs to wipe out data and cause major damage. Perhaps one of the most destructive viruses is called a meme. In his book, *The Virus of the Mind*, Richard Brodie discusses the science of Memetics.

Memetics is the study of memes, or mental viruses. Memes are the equivalent of contagious diseases that infect our thinking. Just like any virus, it is their intention to enter, infect, and spread. A meme is simply a thought passed from one person to another. Most of us catch memes from our parents, teachers, and friends. The memes that have survived have been successful at spreading from person to person and from generation to generation. The vast majority of us continue to spread them today, believing at a subconscious level that the memes are valid and indeed help us. This is essentially what has happened throughout history. We have been programmed to our current way of thinking, and most of us find it difficult, if not impossible, to change. Memes become mental habits. Some memes are good, and some are destructive viruses that infect the mind and place major limitations on individual potential and society as a whole.

Let's see if you're infected. Can you finish this sentence? *Money doesn't grow on …*

How about this one? *Curiosity killed the …*

Don't worry! If you're infected, we will provide you with the antidote for this troublesome type of meme.

The Counter Mindsets

Imagine a series of memes that you believe in your heart and mind to be true. These gems have been passed down from people who love you and care about you. They were packaged as little pearls of wisdom and delivered at just the right times with the intention of helping you learn important lessons. They seem relevant and rational. You even pass them along to your friends and vice versa when the situation calls for a little wisdom. Some of these memes are so powerful that many people share them as if they possessed the sacred keys to happiness and success.

Unfortunately, the memes we're describing have the opposite result. Our research demonstrates that these memes, what we call the *counter mindsets*, lead to lives of frustration, under-performance, and a general sense of mediocrity.

The counter mindsets are best seen in the core lessons experienced in childhood, and it is very likely we will pass them on to our own children, unless there is a conscious intervention. For example, we are all familiar with the saying "Money doesn't grow on trees." When parents use this adage, they are trying to teach their children an important lesson about money. Perhaps they are trying to convey an important connection between hard work, earning, and saving for what you want in life. It is rational thinking, and usually given with the best of intentions. Unfortunately, it's like speaking Italian to someone who only understands English. There is a language barrier, and the parent's intention is usually lost in translation.

When kids hear this saying for the first time, it's probably when they want something special … really badly. They don't like hearing "No," which is what the parents are really saying, but in a sugarcoated way.

When phrases like this are repeated over and over, as parents do when trying to pass along a valuable life lesson, the logic of the lesson is lost and replaced with an emotional scar. Unfortunately, we are inadvertently conditioning our youth into an adversarial relationship with money. Money, in their minds (and later found in the DNA of their habits), becomes seen as a scarce commodity, and a concept that evokes negative emotions. This is why it's not too big a leap to get to the meme, "Money is the root of all evil."

Risky Business

Whether in baseball or business, dating or dominoes, risk is an integral part of success. Taking a chance, especially in the face of potential failure, can be the difference between just surviving and really thriving. Yet here's a meme, a counter mindset we've all heard before, that discourages one of the essential elements of achievement: "Don't make the same mistake twice." When they give this advice, people believe they are teaching children to learn from their mistakes, to continue to grow and expand. When we ask teens what this saying means to them, most say it makes them feel like mistakes are bad. Imagine that Thomas Edison, who failed hundreds of times before finally perfecting the electric light bulb, had embraced that meme.

Perhaps you've heard or used the famous meme, "Curiosity killed the cat." To teens, this means, "Mind your own business." Do we really want to raise kids to not be curious? Where would Albert Einstein and Leonardo da Vinci have been if they had turned off their curiosity switches?

It's not our intention to judge parents and teachers. We believe they're all doing the best they can with the best intentions for their children and students. Consider for a moment the number of times you may have told a child how proud you are of them. It is certainly something we have done hundreds of times. Now consider how the saying, "I am proud of you" may actually teach children to look externally for validation, something we know to be very detrimental. What if simply saying, "You should be proud of yourself" accomplishes everything you want (making the child feel good), but also teaches them to look inside for validation. It really is the subtle language we use every day that is conditioning our children in the very mental habits that are driving lives of struggle and frustration. What if we could change everything, not by making things harder or requiring more information, but rather by adjusting what we are currently doing and saying? And what if that was the difference between an average life and the Ultimate Life?

"Our life is what our thoughts make it."

—Marcus Aurelius

The Scarcity Theory

Henry David Thoreau once said that, "The mass of men live lives of quiet desperation." It is a tragic but very true statement. Statistics show that eighty percent of us do not find fulfillment in our jobs. Current research indicates that depression and suicide are growing at an alarming rate. Experts tell us that more than forty-five percent of marriages end in divorce. The same experts tell us that general discontent continues to grow in society today. Even in a world of ever-expanding opportunity, a growing percentage of us are finding it very difficult to attain joy and fulfillment.

The root of all this suffering is a perception of scarcity. A belief that the world's resources are limited has convinced us that our lives have limitations, too. In truth, humans have lived in a scarce world since the beginning of time. We may have been isolated and alone at times, but despite external scarcities, we thrived. We formed tribes that grew into countries; we developed belief systems that evolved into religions; we took general ideas and expanded them until they became philosophies; and we founded simple systems of bartering and trading that grew into global business communities.

Humans have, throughout our history, gathered in tribes, countries, ethnic communities and religious groups, rather than as a single humanity, thus creating group identities. However, for some, these identities have become more acute and potentially divisive. Many people become disconnected from other individuals and organizations that threaten their identities. In that posture, life becomes a zero sum game. Fear takes over as we fight for our share. We stay in jobs we dislike because we're afraid we won't find new ones, or that one day we'll wake up and find out we don't have enough money. We build relationships based on a need for security rather than meaning and fulfillment. We fight with others over perceived scarcity of resources. We struggle to find happiness, limit our lives, and rarely approach our potential. Perhaps scarcity is just one big meme that we need to release.

We Are Prisoners of Our Five Senses

We live in a world dictated by what we can see, hear, taste, touch, and smell. You're probably familiar with the meme, "Seeing is believing." Is that really true? Our eyes can't see infrared light, yet it does exist. Our human ears can't hear ultrasound, even though a dog can. Current scientific theory maintains that everything in the world that we can experience through one or more of our five senses amounts to only four percent of what actually exists. So everything we can see, hear, etc., like mountains, oceans, cars, clothing and people, adds up to only four percent of what actually exists. This means that ninety-six percent of the world we live in can't be experienced through one of our five senses! This ninety-six percent is often referred to as dark matter. Our five senses limit our view of reality and continue to reinforce our misconception of a world of scarcity. Throughout history, this has been the case. Until the fifteenth century, most people believed the world was flat. This was simply a combination of the way their eyes perceived the visible world and an old belief system that stated the earth was flat. Once the great explorers demonstrated this to be wrong, a whole new world of exploration and trade was created. Similarly, one day Pluto was a planet, and the next day it wasn't.

Life's Window

Along with what we can perceive with our senses, we are also products of our experiences. Our experiences create our reality, as well as our preconceived notions of how the world works when we interact with it. Imagine that, at the instant you're born, you emerge to see a window. The window is clean and wide open. The world is perfect and full of endless possibilities. Then, around age three, you tell your parents you want to learn to fly. They tell you that only birds and bugs can fly, and that humans were made to walk and run. Your dream of flight is squelched, and the shade on the window is lowered just a bit, limiting your view of life.

Later in life, you raise your hand to answer a question in class. You get it wrong, and the teacher is critical, believing you did not do your homework. You think to yourself, "I won't risk that again." So you learn not to take risks, and the window shade lowers a little more. Later in school, you want to try out for a team and your friends tell you that there is no way you'll make the cut. Fearing the ridicule, you don't try out. You want to ask someone on a date, but you tell yourself he or she is out of your league. The window shade lowers and lowers. By the time you are eighteen, ready to go to college and take on the world, you are looking through a two-inch slit of glass, and your view on life's possibilities has shrunk significantly. The world of opportunity you experienced at birth no longer exists through this distorted perspective. It has been reduced to only a fraction of what it might have been had you still believed in your own unique potential. Nothing is different about the world into which you were born … but your perception has changed.

On a Short Rope

In his groundbreaking book *The Four Agreements,* Don Miguel Ruiz discusses how humans are born into a world of unlimited potential. We then go through an experience similar to that of a circus elephant, in which we're trained into a new reality. When an elephant is born, circus trainers tie one end of a rope around the elephant's leg, and the other end to a stake in the ground. The baby elephant is too weak to pull out the stake, and after just a few weeks believes it can't break free and gives up trying. Even as an adult elephant with the strength of dozens of men, the elephant believes it can't break free and doesn't attempt to escape. For the rest of its life, the elephant is contained in a world limited by a stake and a short piece of rope. As happens with most humans, the elephant's world has become the limited place they perceive it to be. The world truly is what we believe it is.

The Subconscious Rules

As our experience and senses provide input into our lives, we develop a set of belief systems rooted in our subconscious minds. These belief systems drive our thoughts and feelings. It is our thoughts and feelings that drive the decisions we make and the actions we take. It is our decisions and actions that determine the results in our lives. Fundamentally, our lives are driven by mindsets that exist at a subconscious level.

The conscious mind can hold about seven pieces of information in short-term memory. The subconscious mind stores everything we have ever learned. *Brain researchers estimate that your unconscious mind outweighs the conscious on a scale of ten million to one.* Science has proven that a subconscious thought travels 800 times faster and is 30,000 times more powerful than a conscious thought. Whether we know it or not, the subconscious mind is far more powerful than the conscious mind. From time to time, our conscious mind will actually come in conflict with our subconscious mind. Now you understand why the subconscious wins when this happens.

Think of yourself as a computer with your conscious mind as the keyboard and monitor. That is where the initiating action takes place, and the computer interacts with the world. The subconscious mind is the underlying software. It simply executes as it is programmed. While the conscious mind (the keyboard) is critical, the ultimate power resides in the subconscious mind or software.

Just as a computer virus can infect an operating system and disrupt all functioning, viruses have infected our minds. They are embedded in our subconscious, driving our feelings and beliefs and, in the end, the decisions we make and the actions we take. We are habitually doing things the same way and expecting different results. Some of us may even try to do things differently with little success, and ultimately fall back into the same behavior patterns. The foundation of personal achievement and the root of happiness and success lie in our mental habits, or mindsets, that have evolved at a subconscious level. It is through them, and only through them, that true life change and increased personal achievement can occur.

Kick the Habit

Our mindsets form habits, and our habits tend to drive the results in our lives. When something in your life is not going the way you want it to go, then you have to make a change. The good news is that many experts believe you can form a new habit in approximately twenty-one days. However, what most people don't realize is that it can take three to six months to change an existing habit, and perhaps even longer depending on how long you've had the habit. This is why so many people fail to make significant changes in their lives, even when they have an idea of what to change. Whether following a diet, a new exercise program, financial advice, or even relationship counseling, you have to stick with it long enough to break the old habits. Most people expect change to happen more quickly and give up too soon, believing that the newfound strategy just isn't working.

Change is hard, no doubt. That is why it is estimated that over ninety-eight percent of personal change efforts fail. Now, however, we have a proven blueprint to the Ultimate Life. The stakes are big, and the rewards tremendous. A true shot at an extraordinary life is the greatest of all end games. Our research, history, and even science is beginning to prove there is a very predictable and repeatable process anyone can undergo to live their dreams. The *7 Mindsets* are the blueprint.

The Incredible Capacity of the Brain

Your brain is the most complex mechanism in the world, and the most influential organ in your body. It has unbelievable capability. In

1997, new camera technology allowed us to view the brain at levels far exceeding anything ever conceived in the past. For the first time, we could view the activity of the brain at a cellular level *while* it was functioning. In one amazing session, it was seen that brain cells have tiny tentacles protruding from them. Each time you perform a function of any kind, these tentacles make connections referred to as DSPs (Dendrite Spinal Protuberances). Smell a flower, and one set of connections is made; blink your eye, and different connections are made. The term scientists have used for this is *plasticity*, meaning that your brain acts like plastic that can be re-formed into an almost infinite set of connections.

With this new knowledge, scientists have estimated the total number of brain cells and the total number of new connections (DSPs) that our brain can make. The number they came up with is staggering. Imagine the number one followed by enough zeroes to fill up an 800-page book. That is a really big number. Now imagine that the last zero went off the last page and was followed by enough 0s to stretch out for 62 million miles. If you can comprehend that number, you can begin to grasp the unbelievable capacity of the human brain. These same scientists have devised a new estimation of our utilization of the brain. They no longer believe that we have tapped into 10 percent of our brain's potential (as was once thought), nor even 1 percent; instead it's more like *1/1,000,000 of a percent*. Simply put, your brain certainly has the capacity to adapt to new mindsets.

Change Your Mindset, Change Your Life

Throughout history, we have gotten bigger, stronger, and faster. Records are broken continually, thus demonstrating the expansion of human potential. Creativity invigorates business, science, and technology, resulting in an ever-expanding realm of possibilities. Some among us accomplish amazing feats and live extraordinary lives. How is it that some people are able to tap into much greater capacities than the rest of us? How are exceptional athletes and musicians able to achieve such high levels of performance? How was Albert Einstein able to develop theories so advanced that most scientists believe we would still not have uncovered them today, one hundred years later? How is Bill Gates able to amass over forty billion dollars in wealth while ninety percent of the world struggles to provide their basic necessities? The answers reside in the mental habits we have and the behaviors they drive in our lives.

The good news is, our research indicates that you can change a mindset and sustain it. By adopting the *7 Mindsets,* you can positively change the outcomes in your life. We will help you do that throughout this book. The next seven chapters will each be devoted to one of the *7 Mindsets*. You will learn to recognize the counter mindsets, and applying the *7 Mindsets* will lead you toward your Ultimate Life. We will guide you every step of the way, and you will be empowered to choose your path.

The Road Less Traveled

Two roads diverged in a wood, and I—
I took the one less traveled by,
And that has made all the difference.

–Robert Frost

The 7 Mindsets to Live Your Ultimate Life

EVERYTHING IS POSSIBLE
PASSION FIRST
WE ARE CONNECTED
100% ACCOUNTABLE
ATTITUDE OF GRATITUDE
LIVE TO GIVE
THE TIME IS NOW

We chose the names for the *7 Mindsets* carefully so young people (and adults, too) could remember them easily. Don't be fooled into thinking that you fully understand the deep meaning behind each Mindset simply by reading its given name. However, once you fully comprehend the explanations we'll provide in the coming chapters, you will find that the simplicity of their names lets you remember them easily and accurately.

Each chapter will include a section called **The Counter Mindsets**. We will describe some of the most common memes that people have inadvertently adopted and which are in direct contradiction to the *7 Mindsets*. This will help you identify and ultimately eliminate them from your subconscious.

Mindsets in Action is a special section in each chapter with specific steps you can take to better learn the *7 Mindsets* and begin activating them in your life.

Lastly, each chapter will conclude with a quick summary called **Mindset in a Minute** to provide you with an unexpected blueprint for an extraordinary life.

Everything Is Possible
Chapter 3

"Risk more than others think is safe. Care more than others think is wise. Dream more than others think is practical. Expect more than others think is possible."
–Claude T. Bissell

The Cornerstone of Modern Motivation

Napoleon Hill was born into poverty and worked his way up from being a young reporter for a small newspaper to being a respected journalist. Hill considered the turning point in his life to have been in 1908, when he was assigned to interview industrialist Andrew Carnegie as part of a series of articles about famous and successful men. Carnegie was one of the richest and most powerful individuals in the world at the time, and Hill discovered that Carnegie believed the process of attaining success could be outlined in a simple formula that anyone could understand and achieve. Impressed with Hill, Carnegie asked if he was up to the task of putting together this information by interviewing or analyzing over 500 successful men and women, many of them millionaires, in order to discover and publish this formula for success.

As part of his research, Hill interviewed many of the most famous people of the time including Thomas Edison, Alexander Graham Bell, George Eastman, Henry Ford, John D. Rockefeller, Sr., Charles M. Schwab, F.W. Woolworth, William Wrigley, Jr., John Wanamaker, William Jennings Bryan, Theodore Roosevelt, and William H. Taft.

Hill's long-term interview-study culminated in one of the greatest books on personal achievement ever written, *Think and Grow Rich*. We believe it to be the preeminent work on dream fulfillment ever conducted. Ultimately, the book came to a rather simple solution, that success is a function of expectations. Hill concluded that the primary predictors of success are 1) having a clear vision for your life, 2) sustaining a burning desire, and 3) expecting to be successful.

"Whatever the mind can conceive and believe it can achieve."

–Napoleon Hill

We have become forecasters of a different source with our years of experience working with schools and youth organizations. When we initially visit a school or organization, we apply our knowledge and powers of observation to make a determination about the environment. One of the things we look for, or to be more precise, what we attempt to feel in our gut, is how much empowerment is in the air.

In schools and organizations that truly empower their students, there is an aura of promise among the youth. There is great clarity in what they want to do with their lives. High expectations are placed on students by their teachers, and the students have high expectations for themselves. After working with over hundreds of thousands teenagers around the world, our research is 100% consistent with that of Napoleon Hill. Our lives are indeed a product of what we expect them to be.

The Final Frontier

Care to go for a ride into outer space? Now you can travel there roundtrip. As part of our research, we interviewed Sir Richard Branson. At the end of the interview, he was asked what he would do differently if he could start over and do it all again. Without hesitation, he responded, "I would dream bigger."

Branson is worth over two billion dollars. He has started more than a hundred companies. He lives on his own private island. Two of his later ventures are Virgin Galactic, the first company to commercialize space tourism, and Virgin Oceanic, which is taking tourists to the deepest points in the Pacific Ocean. Pretty amazing stuff for someone who thinks his dreams aren't big enough.

Branson was not belittling his accomplishments. As a matter of fact, interviews with hundreds of other successful men and women demonstrate that his feelings are shared by most great achievers. When we interviewed Jack Canfield (co-author of *Chicken Soup for the Soul*), he described a survey that asked the most accomplished men and women in the U.S. the same question we asked Branson: "What would you do differently if you could start over?" Their responses were inevitably the same: they would dream bigger, and they would also start sooner.

People like Branson realize that everything which exists in the world today was once just an idea in the mind of an individual curious enough to wonder. Fire, the wheel, electricity, the automobile, the airplane, and the cell phone were all once only in the world of imagination.

But in each case, someone had the idea to bring each from the world of imagination into the real world, making the seemingly impossible possible.

Richard Branson understands that *Everything Is Possible*, and that a clear vision and absolute faith in its possibility will most certainly create a new reality. Once we understand this, as Branson certainly does, we learn that the only limitations in our lives are our own dreams, expectations, and the time we dedicate to making them happen. So why not dream bigger and start now?

The Counter Mindsets

Have you ever watched the movie *Rudy*? If you have, you know the storyline. If you've never seen it, *Rudy* is the story of a young man of average athletic skills who is on the short side, but has a dream of playing for Notre Dame, one of the legendary college football teams in America. Seeking encouragement from one of the priests in the movie, Rudy gets the advice, "The key to happiness is learning to be happy with what you have."

This type of advice is doled out by parents, teachers, and mentors millions of times a day all over the world. It is based on rational thinking and has been passed from generation to generation with one overall intention: to prevent our children from being disappointed. The problem is, advice like this is garbage.

What would Helen Keller's life have been like if she had believed that she needed to learn to be happy with what she had, given her physical limitations? And more importantly, what would Helen's teacher, Anne Sullivan, have believed if she herself had bought into the notion of settling for what was? Together, Helen and Anne proved the world wrong. Anne Sullivan believed it was possible to teach Helen, and she also taught Helen to believe it was possible to learn. Helen lived a full and productive life, becoming one of the most inspirational women to ever live.

How about Wilma Rudolph, who had infantile paralysis when she was young? No one ever expected her to walk, let alone become a super-athlete. Wilma Rudolph became the fastest woman in the world and went on to win three Olympic Gold Medals.

Helen Keller and Wilma Rudolph's lives tell us that the key to happiness is not to settle and be happy with what we've been given, but rather to pursue happiness and believe in what we want.

It is easy to say that Helen Keller and Wilma Rudolph are the exception and not the rule, that they were extraordinary people … and that we're just ordinary. While it's true that Keller and Rudolph emerged as extraordinary women, we should never forget that they began life as less than ordinary, and succeeded because they did not accept low expectations for their lives. Why is it that some achieve extraordinary lives while others struggle? It's because many of us have bought into a limited perception of reality. We are so trapped with what we can see, hear, taste, smell, and touch, that we cannot see or believe in the world of possibilities that awaits us beyond our immediate perceptions.

During World War II, Winston Churchill gave one of his most famous speeches:

> *We shall go on to the end, we shall fight in France, we shall fight on the seas and oceans, we shall fight with growing confidence and growing strength in the air, we shall defend our Island,*

whatever the cost may be, we shall fight on the beaches, we shall fight on the landing grounds, we shall fight in the fields and in the streets, we shall fight in the hills; we shall never surrender, and even if, which I do not for a moment believe, this Island or a large part of it were subjugated and starving, then our Empire beyond the seas, armed and guarded by the British Fleet, would carry on the struggle, until, in God's good time, the New World, with all its power and might, steps forth to the rescue, and the liberation of the old.

In a war that seemed lost, these words changed the expectations of a country and ultimately the world. They shifted the collective consciousness and painted a new vision of the future. Churchill gave his people great hope, and, more importantly, changed their expectations … and the rest is history.

Mindset in Action: A Step-by-Step Approach

Step 1: Look Inside Before You Look Outside

Everything Is Possible is not a naïvely optimistic mindset. It does not mean that a ninety-year-old man can be the MVP of his country's World Cup Soccer team. We are not suggesting that you can be the next great scientist (although you may be) or that you will break the world record in the hundred-yard dash (although you could). When we ask students to share their dreams, most start out with extrinsically-driven dreams like becoming a superstar athlete or rock star. We respond that these dreams may actually happen, but perhaps there is something even better, an expression of their lives that is authentic to who *they* are. For every Lionel Messi, one of the world's best soccer players, there are thousands of schoolteachers who live extraordinary lives of joy and meaning and have an enormous impact. The expressions of their lives are equally as powerful as Oprah Winfrey's or Michael Jordan's. They are achieving what we call their *authentic dreams*, a concept we will dive into more deeply later in the book.

The authentic dream starts deep inside with who you are and what you want. These intrinsic characteristics create the foundation from which you can do what seems impossible. The first step to making everything possible in your life is to stop allowing external factors and influences to define your dreams. Understand what you stand for and what matters to you. When Walt Disney was a young boy, he lived in an idyllic town called Marceline, Missouri. Disney often called it the greatest time of his life. He loved small town culture and often characterized himself as a small town boy. It was a value he would carry with him throughout his life, and a value that came to define much of his work. His found a love for animals in Marceline, which ultimately drove his imagination and his portrayal of animals in his cartoons and feature films. If one visits the Magic Kingdom in Walt Disney World, you can see that Main Street USA and Tom Sawyer Island are modeled after Marceline, Missouri.

Muhammad Ali once defined his primary value as courage; for Mother Teresa it was compassion; for Albert Einstein, curiosity. In addition to being a small town boy, Walt Disney defined himself as a dreamer. You can see how centering with one's core value creates great strength and focus in life, and how it becomes the bedrock of great accomplishments.

Step 2: Challenge Current Thinking

In his book, *How to Think Like Leonardo da Vinci*, Michael Gelb portrays the characteristics of the man some believe to be the greatest genius of all time. One of the seven characteristics that Gelb describes is *Dimostrazione*, an Italian concept meaning, "a constant seeker of truth with a complete lack of willingness to accept any truths other than those one has observed and concluded on his or her own." While most think of art and engineering when hearing the Da Vinci name, his greatest works were in the area of human anatomy. This work is considered by modern scientists to have been 240 years ahead of its time. In Da Vinci's day, the human body was considered a mystical mechanism. Unwilling to accept the then-current dogma, he worked with hundreds of animal and human cadavers to uncover such discoveries as how muscles and tendons work, how blood flows through the body, what the major organs do, and how we breathe air and process food. Only through personal observation and self-discovery did Da Vinci draw the critical conclusions and create the beliefs that formed his thinking.

In his groundbreaking book *The Four Agreements*, Miguel Ruiz talks about the domestication of humans. He claims we are like animals, having been conditioned by our experiences and the collective consciousness of our world. He believes that 999 out of 1,000 people are trapped and that only 1 in 1,000 has managed to break free. He calls these rare people "warriors," being those who continually fight the "parasite" of current mass thinking. In Ruiz's opinion, the path to true freedom and happiness in life requires breaking through the barriers of dogma, challenging all assumptions, and drawing our own conclusions through personal experiences.

Albert Einstein was a pacifist who left Germany because he disagreed with the ideology of the Nazi party. He also unraveled the mysteries of science with theories that challenged the very fiber of our universe.

Martin Luther King, Jr., refused to accept the oppression of others, and Gandhi refused to bow to English Imperialism. Monet and his fellow Impressionists violated the traditional rules of painting and challenged the conventional art community. Elvis Presley, Ray Charles, The Beatles and others changed everything about popular music. The great entrepreneurs and business people of our day have succeeded by creating unique products, processes, and business models. Greatness comes from being different, from looking beyond accepted viewpoints, and by seeking new realms of possibility. This is essential. One must challenge current assumptions and continually try to expand his or her thinking.

Step 3: Engage Your Imagination

Marcus Aurelius is considered one of the five most powerful Roman emperors and possibly the most learned of the Stoic philosophers. Many of his writings were completed on the battlefield as he continually sought greater meaning from life. In one of his classic musings, he stated, "Our lives are dyed with the color of our imagination." What he meant is that our lives, what we achieve, are a product of our ability to envision them.

When most of the world thought computers would never be more than massive mainframes that filled entire floors of buildings, people like Bill Gates and Steve Jobs imagined a computer in every house. When most thought automobiles would only be a luxury of the rich, Henry Ford imagined an assembly line to produce cars for the common man. It is only through our imaginations that we can break out of our current reality. It is impossible to see anything differently if we do not close our eyes and dream a better dream. We must all cultivate a powerful and highly attuned imagination.

In his book, *A Whole New Mind,* Daniel Pink discusses the critical factors of success for the future. In a world of exponential change, we cannot even fathom the world and challenges that will face our children. Pink argues that any routine job will be marginalized and automated. He believes that the imaginative, creative mind will no longer be a luxury, but a necessity for any form of success in the future. Albert Einstein once said, "We cannot solve the problems we face with the same level of thinking that created them." It is only through imagination that we can solve the complex problems we face and deal with the volatile and dynamic nature of the world.

Step 4: Put Your Imagination Into Action

Creativity can be defined as putting our imaginations into action. Seeing a different reality is one thing, but taking action on it is another. Martin Luther King, Jr., had a dream in which his children would be judged by the content of their character, not the color of their skin. It was a big dream with many personal dangers and pitfalls, but he acted on it. He once said, "You do not have to see the entire staircase; you must simply take the first step." King took those steps, because without purposeful and creative action, nothing can change.

Thomas Edison, the American inventor of the light bulb, failed many times when trying to perfect sustainable lighting. When asked how he could keep going, he said, "I have not failed, I've just found 10,000 ways that won't work." Edison, like all celebrated achievers, understood that fantastic accomplishments and notable lives are the culmination of thousands and thousands of tiny steps. Many of the steps (and very likely most of them) are riddled with mistakes, but it is the creative process that is critical.

Look around you. Everything in your life is the product of a creative process. Someone had a dream inspired by their imagination and made it a reality through creative action. We must act on our imaginations and our dreams. We must have the courage to fail, and recognize that every step we take has meaning and is part of the process of reaching our goals.

Step 5: Dream Big! Expect Success, Happiness, and Meaning

We have studied the famous successes, but we have also analyzed the happiest people we know, those people everyone wants to be around and for whom everything always seems to work out. And our consistent conclusion is that they are happy because they expect to be happy. They find meaning because they constantly seek it in every person they meet, every experience they have, and every meal they eat. Happiness and meaning are things they have envisioned all their lives. And expecting happiness is simply another type of dream, a really big dream, if you think about it.

Michelangelo once said, "The greater danger for most of us lies not in setting our aim too high and falling short, but in setting our aim too low and achieving our mark." Like others, he saw a world filled with people who expected too little of themselves and their lives. They saw the lives of their parents and those around them and could never see any further. True happiness and meaning do not come from an absence of failure, but from accomplishment. They come with the expression of one's ability to maximize their potential. As Eleanor Roosevelt once said, "The future belongs to those who believe in the beauty of their dreams."

The vast majority of us have no comprehension of our potential. Recent brain research now demonstrates that we use much less than 1% of our brain's capacity. We are all capable of unbelievably amazing things, but, unfortunately, most of us lock ourselves into a drastically limited view of our world and abilities.

There is a story about actor Jim Carrey, who, while struggling as a new comedian, wrote a check to himself for ten million dollars for acting services rendered. He post-dated the check for ten years later and carried it around in his wallet every day to reaffirm his dream. Almost to the date, ten years later, he found out he was being paid ten million dollars to star in the movie *Dumb and Dumber*. Carrey later became the first actor to receive twenty million dollars for his acting services in one movie.

The happiest and most successful people have higher expectations for their lives. Typically, from an early age, they have a clear and positive image of their future. More importantly, they have the confidence or inner knowledge that they can and will realize their dreams. They may never state it explicitly or even consciously think about it, but when asked later, they always say that they just knew it would happen.

Step 6: Don't Worry About the How

Very few people would take a cross-country road trip without planning ahead. Most likely, they would plan attractions to visit, hotels for lodging, clothes to pack, a budget for meals, and maybe make a playlist for the road. The same can be said about embarking on a new business venture. It's prudent to think and plan ahead to avoid mistakes and increase your odds of success. Perhaps this is why one of the toughest challenges people face is letting go of the *how* when it comes to pursuing their dreams.

Many millionaires went bankrupt before they made their first million.

Home run kings in baseball usually lead the league in strikeouts as well. Failure provides feedback, and the best way to get feedback is to take action. It's okay to create a plan for the pursuit of your dreams, but it is counterproductive to wait until all aspects line up properly, because they never do. They line up along the journey through a maze of trials and tribulations that are impossible to predict. It's only upon achieving a great accomplishment that you can look back and see the perfectly imperfect path that led you to your goal.

It's okay to have confidence in the unknown. Start getting comfortable with ambiguity. In a world where most people are rooted in reality, the path to their dreams is not always clear. Focus on the *what* and the *why*, but don't worry about the *how*. We get so hung up thinking we must have a clear plan, but a plan cannot possibly account for all the creativity and adaptation required to make our dreams a reality. We have to believe in our dreams and our ability to overcome all obstacles along the way. We must be able to recognize the amazing opportunities presented to us each day, opportunities that cannot be envisioned or expected.

In their book *The Passion Test*, Janet Bray Atwood and Chris Atwood use a powerful technique when teaching others to visualize their dreams. When defining a goal or dream, they wrote that we need to identify what it is we think we want and then add "or something better" at the end of the statement. With this simple technique, you can ensure your dreams are never limited by your current reality.

Step 7: Be Wary of Dream Snatchers

The last critical step in making *Everything Is Possible* true in your life is to become vigilant. Our dreams are precious and need to be protected. And we must be vigilant because they often need protection from the people who claim to know what's best for us and also don't want us to become disillusioned or disappointed if our dreams die. We must also be on constant guard against the people who not only dislike our optimism, but are actually jealous of our ability to dream and want nothing more than to shoot our dreams out of the sky.

These dream snatchers often masquerade as friends, but we must be conscious and alert for the negativity a dream snatcher can spread. By recognizing who these dream snatchers are, we can limit their power and not be deterred from our dreams and the actions we must take to achieve them.

He Wishes for the Cloths of Heaven

HAD I the heavens' embroidered cloths,
Enwrought with golden and silver light,
The blue and the dim and the dark cloths
Of night and light and the half-light,
I would spread the cloths under your feet:
But I, being poor, have only my dreams;
I have spread my dreams under your feet;
Tread softly because you tread on my dreams.

−W.B. Yeats

Mindset in a Minute

Everything Is Possible

Dream big, embrace creativity, and expect great results.

Step 1. Look inside before looking outside: Build your life and dreams from a position of strength. Base them on your values and the things that are important to you. From this intrinsically motivated perspective, you will act with courage and sustain the burning desire required for greatness.

Step 2. Challenge current thinking: As soon as you accept another's reality, you have limited your own. Become a seeker of knowledge through your own experiences and see the world from your viewpoint. It is this perspective from which you will build a new reality for your life that extends beyond your current surroundings.

Step 3. Engage your imagination: Train yourself to visualize and see new realities. Never make assumptions about impossibilities; simply have the courage to imagine and believe. It's through our imagination that we start the process of improving on the realities of today.

Step 4. Put your imagination to work through creativity: Build the courage to act on your ideas and dreams. The most powerful actions are purposeful and creative. Only through trial and discovery can we traverse the path to our goals and dreams. We must act on our imagination.

Step 5. Expect success, happiness, and meaning: You must build confidence in your ability to live your dreams, achieve greatness, and most importantly, find happiness and meaning in your life. When you expect these things, you will start to recognize the little things each day that indicate your success. The momentum builds, and your life begins to accelerate in a positive direction toward your goals and dreams.

Step 6. Don't worry about the how: Let go of the need to see exactly how you will make something happen in your life. Often, the required steps cannot possibly be known because they are not part of your current experiences and knowledge base. Have courage in the creative process, and constantly identify and act on opportunities that align with your goals and dreams.

Step 7. **Be wary of dream snatchers:** Be vigilant with your dreams. Understand that they are precious assets. Recognize when they are threatened, and overcome the pressures to let go.

Passion First
Chapter 4

"Many things in life will catch your eye, but only a few will capture your heart—follow those."

—Unknown

The Seed of Life

If money didn't matter, what would you do for free? How would you spend your days? What business would you start? What career would you pursue? What would fill your life with joy? When we speak to teenagers, they easily answer these questions, although usually their first responses involve wanting to become superstar athletes, rock stars, celebrities, and mega-mogul zillionaire entrepreneurs. College students have a little more trouble answering, as the answers often seem in direct conflict with the major they're pursuing or the job interviews they have lined up. Most adults, frankly, are stymied by these questions. It's as if the part of their brain that once dreamed of such wonderful things has become dormant. It's no wonder that, according to a major Gallup Survey, approximately eighty percent of adults say that they aren't passionate about what they do for a living.

Imagine for a moment that you are born with a special and unique seed inside of you. You might think of it as your *soul seed* or *passion seed*. Throughout your life, this seed evolves, and growing with it is your unique calling. You can choose to ignore it or perhaps only care for it on the weekend. But it will not go away. You will constantly be reminded of who you are capable of becoming. Many adults experience a mid-life crisis, a time in their lives when they pause and ask, "Is this all there is? Is this why I'm here?" The mid-life crisis doesn't discriminate. It hits the affluent, who wonder why money hasn't bought them true happiness; and it hits people who are struggling, forcing them to wonder if they settled too often in life. These are times to re-examine your life and the choices you made, to consider starting over with greater purpose, and to listen to your passion seed ... finally!

The Quarter-Life Crisis

According to authors Alexandra Robbins and Abby Wilner, there is now such a thing as a quarter-life crisis affecting young people in their twenties. Here's a remarkable depiction from one of their readers:

I have always referred to this time in my life as my "mid-twenties" crisis. Everyone I know that's my age is in it unless they majored in business or computer-related subjects and got a dream job right out of college. The rest of us are floating around aimlessly trying to find a niche. An undergrad degree is worthless most of the time, and so we end up in dead-end jobs we aren't happy in. We question our dreams, we wonder if we are settling or giving up, we consider whether we should still carry our dreams or just let them remain "dreams." It's hard to decipher whether or not reality is "giving up" or reality is just plain reality. Then again, you hear about people like Mozart, Britney Spears, and Jesse Jackson and other people in this world achieving their "impossible" dreams ... and you wonder if it is blind luck on their part, or if they just did something we haven't figured out yet.

There's no need to wonder anymore. Our research clearly indicates that finding your passion and organizing your life around who you're meant to be is the clearest path to living your dreams. In a recent interview that ended her talk show's twenty-five-year run, Oprah Winfrey commanded that we follow our passions, for if we do not, we can never be truly happy.

To Be or Not to Be

William Shakespeare once wrote, "This above all else, to thine own self be true." Perhaps no more powerful a statement has ever been made, for true happiness is found when we find our authentic selves. Lao Tzu is the author of the *Tao Te Ch'ing*. It is believed by many that Lao Tzu was a records keeper who maintained the spiritual teachings of the Eastern masters from China in the 6th Century BCE. The Tao, therefore, was the culmination of one of the most prolific periods of enlightenment in history. In one passage from his powerful work, he states, "At the center of your being you have the answer; you know who you are and you know what you want." Lao Tzu later wrote, "To know others is wisdom; to know yourself is enlightenment." Science has proven that we are unique, that no one has ever existed like us or ever will exist. We are each a completely unique expression of human life. Our purpose is to find our unique genius, build the courage to pursue it, and share that genius with the world to the maximum extent possible.

"The two greatest days in your life are the day you are born and the day you discover why."

—William Barclay

The Counter Mindsets

In the movie *Jerry McGuire,* there is a scene in which actor Cuba Gooding, Jr., forces his agent, played by Tom Cruise, to yell "Show me the money!" A professional football player, Cuba wants validation of his talent in the form of a large contract with a top-tier team. This mindset is rooted in the very fiber of the free world: an extrinsically-driven motivation that views wealth creation as life's true measuring stick. On many occasions, all of us make decisions that put money first, relegating our intrinsic characteristics and desires to a secondary role.

Common advice young people receive when choosing a college, selecting a major, and even applying for a job is to think of the future opportunities that their choice will provide. Which college will help set them up for a good job? What subjects will prepare them for broader career options? Which job offers more money, better benefits, and room for growth? These are all rational thoughts, but according to our research, they are the wrong questions to ask. Putting money first is almost always the path to a life devoid of real passion and lowered expectations.

Instead of putting money first, lead with what you would do for free. What subjects and pursuits give you the greatest joy? What work inspires you? What comes easy to you and is difficult for others? The intersection of your passions and your talents will get you started on the path to an extraordinary life. People who put their passions first tend to work harder than those who don't love what they do. Those with passion learn more, put in the extra time (not because they have to, but because they *want* to), become experts in their fields, are more enjoyable to be around, and are determined to hang in there when times get tough. That's why the ultra successful all say that when they followed their passions, they ended up making more money than they thought was possible. The joke is on everyone else, though, because most of them admit that they would have done their work for free.

There is a saying: "In life, you can choose either security or freedom, and if you choose security, you will have neither." Too many of us are giving up our dreams in pursuit of the unattainable. We have researched numerous folks who possess tremendous wealth, and the common thread is that money will not make you happy. What makes a person happy is the most fundamental currency: meaning in life. Money can facilitate attaining access and accumulating goods, but money should never be the primary driving force. Happiness comes from doing what you love, with people you love doing things with, and getting a great sense of accomplishment and meaning from what you do. People chase success when it's significance they really seek. When you put your *Passion First*, then true happiness is the journey, not the destination.

Passion, in addition to being based on your personal interests, is also rooted in what matters to you. If done right, your goals and dreams should drive the results you want in life. In other words, the fruits of your passionate labor must create things and impact people that matter to you in a profound manner. No matter what your chosen vocation, great success and meaning will require overcoming massive hurdles and obstacles along the way. If the results do not matter enough to you, somewhere along the way you will stop, and the dream will never be fulfilled.

Mindset in Action: A Step-by-Step Approach

Step 1: Play to Your Strengths

Aristotle was the student of Plato and the teacher of Alexander the Great in ancient Greece. He, along with Plato and Socrates, are the primary drivers of the "Greek Miracle," the philosophy that transitioned Western society from believing in mythology to rational thinking. Along with his student, Alexander the Great, scholars consider Aristotle to be one of the most brilliant minds who ever lived. Very few, if any, of equivalent intelligence have studied human nature and achievement at the level of Aristotle. Our favorite of his teachings is summed up in his quote, "Where the needs of the world and your talents cross, therein lies your vocation." What Aristotle taught us over 2,300 years ago was a pretty straightforward concept of playing to your strengths.

In his book, *Now Discover Your Strengths*, Marcus Buckingham describes a culture of focusing on and minimizing our weaknesses. Supported by extensive research, his position is that corporations focus on training to help their employees overcome their shortcomings. Buckingham urges our schools and organizations to instead become strength-based, and leverage individuals' strengths to achieve maximum success and productivity.

Howard Gardner, a developmental psychologist, is critical of our school systems, which currently teach and assess our students in only two primary categories of intelligence (linguistic and logical/mathematical). In his *Theory of Multiple Intelligences*, he argues that there are nine areas in which individuals can excel (he adds spatial, kinesthetic, musical, inter- and intra-personal, naturalistic, and existential). Sir Ken Robinson, author of the bestselling book *The Element*, agrees with Gardner that the current state of education is systematically eliminating much of the true talent that exists in our youth. He jokingly debates Gardner, saying there are far more than nine intelligences, more like billions, or the equivalent of the current number of people on our planet.

The Johnson O'Connor Foundation is a leader in helping youth and adults uncover their natural talents and abilities. While most people look for obvious strengths such as math, music, art, or athletics, the Johnson O'Connor assessment goes much deeper. They look not only at the most obvious aptitudes, but seek a deeper understanding of one's talents. They seek to answer questions like, "in what type of situations does one perform best?" and, "with what types of people does one work the best?" It is this type of understanding that truly allows one to attain optimum achievement. What time of day are they the most creative? Are they good under pressure or do they need harmony? Do they accomplish more in groups or alone? We must attain this level of understanding in ourselves before we can truly unleash our potential to its fullest. Learn to identify your strengths, and search for ways to improve them and align them with your daily life.

Step 2: Pursue Your Passions

In his great book, *The Alchemist,* Paulo Coelho tells the story of a young boy on a journey to discover his "Personal Treasure." The personal treasure was, essentially, the boy's reason for living, the purpose of his life, rooted in that which mattered to him and about which he was passionate. It is a very simple concept, known and passed down for thousands of years. Greatness and genius are the offspring of one's ability to focus. Albert Einstein once said, "It is not that I am more intelligent, it is only that I am passionately curious." It was a consuming desire to understand, not his genius, which guided Einstein to revolutionize our understanding of the universe. His ability to focus on the problem came from a deep-rooted passion to solve it. If you want to achieve greatness, you must align with your passion. It is passion that will motivate you to do all the things required for greatness. You will read more, practice more, learn from others more, and achieve more. Those are the means by which your life will gain deeper meaning.

Finding your passion is an extremely introspective process. It requires trial and error, and the constant building of a deeper awareness of oneself. We would argue that it is a never-ending process because your wants, needs, and desires are always evolving. The important thing is that you seek to identify your passion, and then pursue it with courage. If you think you are passionate about making music, take a guitar or piano lesson and find out. If you find that cooking food is something you enjoy, see if you can take it to the next level by working at a restaurant or preparing extravagant meals for guests in your home. Every day of your life should be a constant pursuit of your own "Personal Treasure."

Step 3: Connect Your Uniqueness to the World Around You

The story of Bill Gates is described by Malcolm Gladwell in his book, *Outliers*. Gates and his counterpart, the late Steve Jobs, founder of Apple, were the primary catalysts of the computer and software revolutions. Both were extremely intelligent, and both had a true passion for emerging technology. What drove their success was timing. They both happened to be twenty-five years old in 1980. At that time, technology was ready for a revolution. What was needed was someone young enough to be progressive in his thinking, yet mature enough to understand the practical realities of business. Gates and Jobs both fit that profile, and the rest is history. Each enjoyed overwhelming success connected to his unique genius, but equally critical was how they applied their intellects.

Throughout history, the most significant triumphs have been a product of timing. Nelson Mandela and Gandhi each appeared during a time when his country and its people were ready for and very much in need of social change. Martin Luther King was there when Rosa Parks decided not to move to the back of the bus. Abraham Lincoln led our nation through the Civil War, and Anne Frank's presence in an attic transformed our understanding of the Holocaust. Michelangelo gilded the Renaissance, and Mother Teresa served an impoverished India.

We must look inside to uncover our own unique genius, but we must look outside to understand how to impact the world in the most positive manner. This takes courage, because you may be treading on new ground. The world may not initially receive you with open arms. People like what is familiar, and often reject new ideas. Early focus groups hated the search engine name Google, simply because it was foreign to them. Now it's not only a household name, but also a verb. Automotive innovator Henry Ford once commented that if he'd asked his potential customers what they wanted, they would've said, "a faster horse." Be a pioneer as you look to connect your unique genius to the world around you.

Step 4: Build Your Authentic Dreams

People often criticize the leaders of the American Industrial Revolution as tyrants. John D. Rockefeller, J. P. Morgan, Andrew

Carnegie, and others are often portrayed as greedy individuals who accumulated great wealth at the expense of others. Studies of these individuals show there are certainly aspects of their lives and character that one could question. However, what cannot be questioned are their achievements and their unwavering commitment to succeed. All these men had more money than they needed, and most gave all of it away to charities. The ultimate driving force for each of them was the impact their monopolies would have on the world. Cornelius Vanderbilt, for example, believed nothing was more important than an interconnected network of railroads that would facilitate trade and spawn economic growth. The vision and dream of this was at the very fiber of his existence. It was of the utmost importance. The same can be said about J. P. Morgan and banking, Andrew Carnegie and steel, Rockefeller and oil, or Henry Ford and the automobile.

You will hear people say that nothing comes easy. It is true that whatever your endeavor in life, there will be complexities and challenges along the way. For legendary basketball player Michael Jordan, his obstacle was the Detroit Pistons. For three years they had beaten his team, the Chicago Bulls, in the playoffs and gone on to the championship. John Daly, the coach of the Pistons, had devised a special defense solely to stop Jordan. In *The Jordan Rules* by Sam Smith, the author details a defense that basically beat Jordan up for four quarters. Jordan responded with greater determination. He rebuilt his physique and became stronger. He developed an outside shot, and his team defeated the Pistons in 1991 and went on to win the NBA title.

You must develop authentic dreams; these are visions and goals that matter most to you, and that you believe are of the highest importance. It may be the development of your children, or it could be an NBA championship. The point is, the only way to overcome all the obstacles and challenges you'll encounter is for the dream to matter enough to give you the courage, motivation, and tenacity to persevere. Actor Will Smith believes that you need to find a purpose so important that you are willing to die for it. It has to matter *that much* for you to make it happen. Real passion comes from pursuing authentic dreams that burn like a raging fire inside you.

Step 5: Lean Into Your Passion

In their book, *The Passion Test*, the authors suggest making decisions in favor of what you're passionate about. When deciding between two jobs, choose the one that is more closely aligned with your passion. Trying to decide what class to take? Choose in favor of your passion. Looking to start a business? Before you do, think about what you are most passionate about. Scott's brother, Jadd, is passionate about music. He went on a music-related job interview and thought it was a perfect match. Then he learned that the company didn't have money to hire anyone at that point and was only doing some preliminary research. Scott suggested that if Jadd really liked the opportunity, then perhaps he could volunteer some of his time. The rationale was that at least he would be surrounding himself with people and work about which he was passionate. Scott told him not to worry about the money and to just have fun.

One day while Jadd was volunteering, an opportunity came up for him to shoot a music video with his band, something he had always wanted to do. Not only did he find out about this opportunity because he was volunteering that day, but the video was produced at almost no cost because it was part of a contest. Jadd was in the right place at the right time. Is this a coincidence, or is it the natural by-product of leaning into your passion? It's important to remember that when you lean in, you must do so with both eyes open for opportunities to continue choosing in favor of your passion.

Step 6: Embrace Your Destiny

In his book, *The Seven Spiritual Laws of Success*, Deepak Chopra introduces the concept of Dharma, an ancient Sanskrit term that epitomizes the meaning of the *Passion First* Mindset. Inside each of us is a *soul seed*, a boundless capacity, and a wonderful gift to share. Our primary purpose in life is to search within ourselves and uncover this unique genius, then express and share it with the world. It is through our Dharma that we will create the most value with our lives and derive the most joy and meaning in return. We must uncover the soul seed and nurture it. If we can do this, we will reap a lifetime of joy and bliss.

This joy and bliss do not come without some cost. We must sustain the courage to act on our destiny. At times, that may mean suffering or being ridiculed. Through your self-discovery process, you may find your unique genius is not what you thought you wanted. It may not fit in or be cool. It may challenge current thinking or be resisted by others. The people you love may not agree with you and might try to persuade you to go in other directions. To be great, we must be different, and different is not always comfortable.

Every story of success and happiness contains challenge, risk and adversity. Bill Gates dropped out of Harvard to pursue his dream. It is doubtful that many felt that was in his best interest. Abraham Lincoln saw his country suffer around his purpose of preserving a single, unified nation. People laughed at Wilma Rudolph who, as a crippled young girl, talked of becoming the fastest woman in the world. Pursuing your passion requires you to make difficult decisions, ones that align with your authentic dreams and might push other pursuits or relationships to the side. Often, decisions you make that align with your passion may not seem financially sound. How you will support yourself and provide the basic necessities of life might be a concern. The point is, you must trust your genius. Relish the uncertainty, knowing you can and will succeed. Embrace your destiny, and be fully committed to doing whatever it takes to pursue your passion.

"Do not wish to be anything but what you are, and try to be that perfectly."
—St. Francis of De Sales

Mindset in a Minute

Passion First

Pursue your authentic talents and deepest interests.

Step 1. Play to your strengths: You will be much more successful doing things at which you excel. This also means putting yourself in situations and environments in which you thrive, and with people who bring out the best in you. Understand your strengths, and align what you do with where you can create the most value.

Step 2. Pursue your passions: You can only achieve greatness doing things in which you are interested. Through your passion, you will sustain the focus and do what needs to be done to overcome obstacles and achieve greatness. Identifying and pursing your passions is a lifelong journey!

Step 3. Connect your uniqueness with the world around you: Your talents and passions can only be utilized if they are put into action that creates value. Constantly seek out ways to apply your abilities and interests in the world to create value.

Step 4. Build your authentic dreams: With an understanding of your unique genius and the needs of the world, redefine your dreams. Make sure the outcomes of those dreams are of the most critical importance to your life. If your dreams matter enough to you, this will be the fuel to overcome the obstacles and challenges you'll face.

Step 5. Lean into your passions: When you are confronted with a difficult decision, weigh the options and choose in favor of your passion. It's never too soon or too late to start pursuing your passions. Dreams have no expiration date.

Step 6. Embrace your genius: You must find great satisfaction in who you are and what your life is all about. Embrace your destiny, and trust your genius to move forward toward the life of your dreams.

"What lies behind us and what lies before us are tiny matters compared to what lies within us."

–Ralph Waldo Emerson

We Are Connected
Chapter 5

"If you can accomplish your dream alone, you aren't dreaming big enough."
                                                        –Scott Rigsby

I Was Just Thinking About You!

Have you ever experienced the phenomenon of thinking about a friend or family member you haven't seen or spoken with in a long time, then within hours or days, they call you, seemingly out of the blue? We ask this question to hundreds and thousands of people in large presentation rooms and are always amazed at how many raise their hands. We researched various scientific reasons for this, and some of what we uncovered is mind-boggling, from *quantum entanglement* to *the DNA phantom effect*. However, this book is about mindsets, and sometimes you just need to lean into a mindset long enough to experience the personal evidence for yourself.

In the case of the above-mentioned phenomena, there appears to be something going on that, for now, we'll call *We Are Connected*. At its core, this mindset is about learning to work with, for, and through others to create better lives. In reality, it goes much deeper than that, because it addresses all our relationships, from those characterized by a deep and permanent bond to those that may even seem casual and meaningless.

This chapter will show you how to leverage this unique connection to others.

In his book, *The Butterfly Effect*, Andy Andrews, a New York Times bestselling author and expert on personal achievement, talks about being very curious why some people can just never catch a break. According to them, their lives are in the pits, and it just seems to get worse and worse. Andy jokingly says, "They're right!" He then compares these hapless individuals to other people we all know whose lives always turn up roses. Good things seem to be attracted to them, and their lives just get better and better. Andy then repeats "And they are right!" After years of study, Andy believes the answer to his question is very simple: *"People living great lives are the types of folk that others want to be around. They constantly make positive and meaningful connections, and they use relationships to constantly expand their own happiness and success."*

Everyone who comes into our lives has a skill, a unique perspective, or a piece of knowledge that is essential to fulfilling our dreams. Next time you meet someone, test it out. Deliberately engage this person in a conversation to find out how he or she can help you live your dreams. It could be something as small as them knowing someone who can help you fix a leaky faucet, or it could lead to a deep connection with someone that could ultimately prove life-changing, such as connecting you with critical business partners or a companion. We believe you will find the reason your paths crossed; and the synergy, if leveraged, will take you a step closer to your

Ultimate Life.

The Counter Mindsets

You've probably heard the expression, "It's a dog-eat-dog world," implying that we are in direct competition with one another. Perhaps you can remember a parent, teacher, or friend telling you, "If you want something done right, you have to do it yourself." Over a short period of time, we all seem to have built a world where perceived strength comes from complete independence and autonomy. To be a *self-made man* is considered a great compliment. While the outcome (achieving our goal) might be beneficial, the path to success does not have to be one of solitude. In fact, our research proves that those who have achieved extraordinary success have emphatically stated that they couldn't have done it alone.

We are truly connected, and it is those connections in our lives that help us follow our individual paths. Going it alone might seem to be more courageous, but so much time can be wasted if we isolate ourselves and fail to see how much further we can go if we just reach out.

There's no denying that life can be tough. M. Scott Peck, the author of the mega-selling book, *The Road Less Traveled,* begins by telling his readers that life is difficult. How much more difficult do we make it when we don't tap into the wealth of positive life experiences being offered to us from others if we only take the time to make connections?

Mindset in Action: A Step-by-Step Approach

Step 1: Create a Sense of Connectedness

The first step to living the *We Are Connected* Mindset is the most difficult but also the most essential. Too many of us today feel alone. We have isolated ourselves from others and the world around us. Michael Gelb, the Leonardo da Vinci historian, describes interconnectedness as one of Da Vinci's defining qualities, and one that was instrumental to his success. Leonardo was one of the first "system" thinkers. His passion for anatomy was driven by the curiosity to understand how all the body's organs work together to create and support life. Da Vinci was a strong believer in the concept of "Yin and Yang," a concept from Chinese philosophy which holds that polar opposites and seemingly contrary forces are interconnected and interdependent throughout the natural world. One commonly held belief is that the Mona Lisa was Da Vinci's favorite painting, precisely because it embodied the perfect harmony of humanity and nature.

The first step is to lean into the feeling that there is deeper meaning in all relationships and in all things around the world. The greater sense of connectedness you'll feel can then inspire you to seek out synergies and meaning in all your relationships. It might help if you lean in to the feeling that everything happens for a reason, and everyone comes into our lives for a reason. This will help you view all experiences with a heightened sense of awareness and look to squeeze much more meaning and joy from your life.

Step 2: Choose Empowering Relationships

In his book *The Art of Exceptional Living*, Jim Rohn said, "You are the average of the five people you spend the most time with."

Statistically speaking, folks who are unhappy hang out with unhappy people. People who struggle financially spend most of their time with others who are struggling. People who get divorced very likely have friends or family members who are divorced. Birds of a feather do flock together. Consider closely those with whom you spend your time. Always consider what influences they have on you, and whether they're building you up or breaking you down. Are your friends and coworkers empowering you or bringing you down? Are you empowering them to live their best lives? Think how inspirational it would be to have a close circle of people regularly supporting and empowering one another to greater levels of achievement and joy.

Step 3: Embrace Competition

In 2009, Tiger Woods was competing with Padrig Harrington in the Bridgestone Invitational golf tournament. At the time, Tiger was number one in the world; and Harrington was considered by many to be the number one contender to the throne. The tournament came down to the final nine holes, and everyone prepared for an amazing competition between golf's two best players. On the sixteenth hole, Woods trailed by one shot. A notoriously slow player, Harrington was warned by the officials that if he did not speed up play, he would be penalized. Uncharacteristically, Harrington became flustered and made a triple bogey on the hole, essentially handing the tournament to Woods.

After the tournament, Woods was interviewed. The reporter asked Tiger about the back nine and competing with Harrington. Visibly frustrated, Woods criticized the actions that were taken against Harrington in an effort to speed up his slow play on the sixteenth hole. What frustrated Woods the most was the lost opportunity for him to compete at the very highest level with one of the best golfers in the world.

Regardless of Tiger Wood's lifestyle, no one denies how dominant he was at his craft for over a decade. Many, including most golfers, consider him the greatest golfer ever as well as one of the most talented athletes to ever play any sport. Most of us would have been thrilled with an easy victory. Sure, we might have felt a little sorry for Harrington, but deep down, we would be ecstatic that we won the trophy and took home the big check.

Athletes like Tiger Woods and Michael Jordan see competition differently. For them, competition is the catalyst to greatness. It is only through playing with the best at their best that they can ultimately become better; and only by becoming better can they truly feel the great sense of meaning that we all desire. Tiger Woods saw the competition with Padrig Harrington as an opportunity, but not to get a trophy or win some money. It was an opportunity to learn something about himself, and to become a better golfer by pushing himself to do his very best under the most stressful circumstances.

Step 4: Relish Diversity

In her book *Team of Rivals,* Doris Kearns Goodwin tells the story of Abraham Lincoln and a number of political adversaries he defeated in the 1860 presidential election. Lincoln's venomous political adversaries Edward Bates, Salmon P. Chase and William H. Seward didn't fade from view after the election. Instead, Lincoln appointed his opponents to the cabinet level positions of Attorney General, Secretary of the Treasury, and Secretary of State. While most newly elected presidents would have banished their adversaries, Lincoln understood the great genius these men possessed. Further, he recognized how their numerous political strengths would be vital as he led the country into Civil War.

Instead of separating from his adversaries, Lincoln invited each to join his cabinet. What followed were some of the most intense and heated discussions any president has ever endured. But what ultimately resulted were decisions and a collective fortitude that saved the Union and kept the United States *united.*

Too often, we identify ourselves with a group or a way of thinking. Once it becomes part of our identity, we resist other groups or ways of thinking because we believe they threaten the very fiber of who we are. Da Vinci once said, "I do not care that I am right; what I care about is getting the right answer." That is the essence of what embracing diversity means. We suggest you relish different viewpoints and perspectives and have healthy constructive debates. This may help you come to conclusions and decisions that will be much more effective than the ones you would reach on your own.

Step 5: Build Your Dream Team

Author Andy Andrews says, "All opportunities and new knowledge come through others." Imagine believing that everyone you come in contact with in your life is critical to helping you live your dreams. Knowing this, you would enter every encounter and relationship with a heightened sense of energy and preparedness. People would find greater joy in being around you. Your interactions would become richer and your relationships more meaningful. You would consistently seek and find synergies with others. You would constantly find new opportunities and gain knowledge that you previously might have missed. Your life would become richer in every way.

In Andrews' book *The Seven Decisions*, he talks about creating your own personal board of directors, a group of people you surround yourself with who have expertise in areas in which you need help. Your best friend may be a really good father who is willing to mentor you on parenting. Your financial advisor is the person you go to for financial advice. You may have a personal trainer who helps you with a diet and exercise plan. Even if you don't hire people to fill these roles, you can find people with whom you are friends to serve as unofficial mentors. What Andrews calls "Your Personal Board of Directors," we call "Your Dream Team."

Life can be complicated, with many moving parts that must be managed to live your Ultimate Life. No one was born with the wisdom to effectively manage career, marriage, family, finances, and health. We all need help, and we are surrounded by people with information and knowledge that can make a difference in our lives. Our good friend and business partner Mitchell Schlimer has termed this *OPE,* or *Other People's Experiences*. We must leverage the experiences and knowledge of others as a foundation and launching point for the lives of our dreams.

Step 6: Always Seek Synergies

Walt Disney is considered one of the finest producers in the entertainment industry. It can be argued that no one has achieved his level of success and pushed an industry further. From the first film with synchronized sound to Disney World, his life embodied dreaming big and doing the impossible. For the first half of his career, Walt made a living producing films for movie theatres. When TV was introduced, it was a real threat to his livelihood. As a matter of fact, all the major film studios fought the new medium vehemently.

Walt Disney, however, sought to embrace television. He once said, "TV was not the enemy of the studios, but rather the ally." For him it became another way to distribute his products. What many people do not realize is that it was TV that actually enabled Walt to build Disneyland in California. At the time, ABC was the smallest of the three networks, lagging behind NBC and CBS. ABC was looking for new content that could reposition them and put them on a path of growth. Walt structured a deal to bring Disney programming to ABC, and gained an investment from them that actually allowed Disneyland to be constructed. The rest, as they say, is history. Moreover, the Disney brand and its famous front men, Walt Disney and Mickey Mouse, received critical exposure through television that propelled the Disney brand into becoming one of the most powerful in the world today.

In his book, *The 21 Irrefutable Laws of Leadership*, John Maxwell describes a period of great stress in the life of John Schnatter, the founder of Papa John's Pizza. Schnatter had grown Papa John's to a fairly large pizza delivery business, but his life was a mess. He was stressed out and working ridiculous hours. In a cold sweat, Schnatter woke one morning with a clear realization. He concluded that he was unable to work any harder or any smarter than he was already working. Until he learned to work through others, his life would always be drastically limited. He changed his entire management philosophy, letting go of control and empowering others to help him build the business. Today, Papa John's operates 3,500 restaurants located throughout all 50 states in the U.S. and in 29 countries.

Every person who comes into your life can help you live your dreams. But it's up to you to find the synergy with them yourself—the mutual benefit that will help create better lives for each of you, and ultimately a better world. It's essential that you learn to effectively work with, for, and through others; because they can give you new knowledge and opportunities, provide you with critical talents and skills, and have an exponentially positive impact on the meaning of your life.

Step 7: Seek to Serve First

Author, businessman, and motivational speaker Zig Ziglar is famous for saying, "You can get everything you want out of life if you simply help enough others get what they want." As it relates to the *We Are Connected* Mindset, no truer words have ever been spoken. As previously mentioned, almost all new knowledge and opportunities come through other people. So the question is, how do we best tap into those opportunities? The simple answer is to figure out what you can do to help them.

Remember, everyone who comes into your life can help you live your dreams. You must seek this out, and the best way to do so is to ask how *you* can help *them*. Create a dialogue that searches for the synergies in your new or expanding relationship. Once these synergies are found, the process of co-creation is maximized.

"Alone we can do so little; together we can do so much."

–Helen Keller

Mindset in a Minute

We Are Connected

Explore the synergies in all relationships and learn to empower one another.

Step 1. Create a sense of connectedness: The first step is to feel a sense of interconnectedness with others. This provides the foundation on which to build meaningful, synergistic relationships.

Step 2. Choose empowering relationships: Seek friendships and work associates with the intention of helping each other live lives of greater meaning and significance.

Step 3. Relish competition: Get excited by competition, knowing that its primary purpose is to heighten your own performance and drive you to become better.

Step 4. Celebrate diversity: Be proud of your unique genius, but also find beauty in the diversity of all people. Understand the incredible contributions that people who are different from you can offer.

Step 5. Build your Dream Team: Recognize all the people in your life that you can tap into for guidance and support to maximize your potential and live your dreams.

Step 6. Always seek synergies: Actively seek synergies with everyone you meet, finding how you are able to assist and leverage one another to collective new heights.

Step 7. Seek to serve first: Jumpstart all relationships by focusing first on what you can give or do to help others.

"The most important single ingredient in the formula of success is knowing how to get along with people."

–President Theodore Roosevelt

100% Accountable
Chapter 6

"If it is to be, it is up to me."

–William H. Johnsen

Do You Believe in Magic?

Earvin "Magic" Johnson is considered one of the greatest basketball players to ever play the game. Many experts also believe he was the game's finest point guard. His ability to pass the ball and involve his teammates was unparalleled, and more importantly, that ability helped his team to succeed. Over the course of his career, his 10,141 assists earned him one of the top rankings in the basketball record book. However, even though his career was shortened due to illness, his average of 11.9 assists per game continues to rank number one and positions him as the best passer of all time.

In one game, with seconds left on the clock, Magic made a pass to a rookie teammate who was unable to catch the ball and fumbled it out of bounds. They lost the game. When interviewed after the game, Magic was asked about the pass and if he was frustrated that the young player was unable to catch it and make the basket. Magic's response was that it was a bad pass. The interviewer challenged him by saying it was perfect, the ball hit the player in the hands, and there was no reason he should have dropped it. Magic simply said, "Any pass I make that is not caught is a bad pass." He went on to explain that he knew the young player was nervous, and he was not mentally ready to catch the hard pass under all that pressure. Magic said under those circumstances he should have taken the shot himself.

Magic Johnson's thought process embodies the *100% Accountable* Mindset. Certainly, the rookie should have caught the pass, but the only thing Magic could have done to prevent the ball from being dropped was not to pass the ball to him in the first place. He could have easily placed the blame on his teammate and assumed the role of victim, as the vast majority of players would have done. Instead, he decided on accountability and assessed what he needed to do differently the next time. Magic chose to learn and evolve, and that is a large reason why he is arguably the greatest point guard in the history of basketball.

The Counter Mindsets

Have you heard people say, "just my luck" when something doesn't go their way? How about, "I'd rather be lucky than good." Buying into these perspectives can be very dangerous. Unfortunately, many people walk around feeling like they have very little control over the circumstances in their lives. From a Mindset perspective, this can lead to a *victim* mentality. Once we start blaming other people and events for our situations in life, we become more likely to stop looking for ways to improve and change our future outcomes. For many people, this leads to getting stuck in a rut and repeating the same set of circumstances over and over again. This validates what Albert

Einstein once said: "Insanity is doing the same thing over and over and expecting different results."

Once we stop looking in the mirror for responsibility, we lose control and become victims of our own thinking. We lack the perspective of ancient Roman philosopher Lucius Annaeus Seneca, who once said, "Luck is what happens when preparation meets opportunity." This is the mindset that people of profound happiness and success buy into. The ultra successful understand that they may not be able to control all the events in their life, but they can control how they react to them. They also understand that how they react to events influences what happens next. When you fully embrace this mindset, the effects are liberating. You learn to appreciate that only you control the keys to your happiness and success. By following the suggested Mindset in Action steps, you can move from victim to victor.

Mindset in Action: A Step-by-Step Approach

Step 1: Reconcile with the Past

In the movie *Forrest Gump*, actor Gary Sinise plays Lieutenant Dan, a bitter soldier who lost his legs in the Vietnam War. In the years following the war, Lieutenant Dan is deeply angry and highly focused on the unfairness of his disability. He becomes an alcoholic and watches his life unravel as he spirals out of control. In one scene, while on a shrimp boat stuck in a hurricane, Dan climbs to the highest mast on the ship and fights the hurricane with all his bitterness and anger. The next day, when the hurricane has passed, Forrest Gump finds Dan swimming in the water at complete peace. Somehow, during the night, he had fought off all his demons and reconciled with all the past transgressions against him. Lieutenant Dan was now prepared to move forward with his life. He decided to get artificial limbs and marry a woman from Vietnam. He reconciled his past and removed the mental baggage holding him back.

There is a Buddhist saying that illustrates this point: "Pain is inevitable, but suffering is optional." The problem most of us have when bad things occur is that we continue to relive them over and over again. They take over our lives, make us bitter, and channel our energy away from what we need to do to achieve the happiness and success we all want. It's extremely hard to let go of anger, but we must realize that it's only hurting us and find a way to reconcile and free ourselves from the past so we can effectively move forward. Remember that forgiveness begins and ends with you, and the pain you dwell on is only hurting you.

Step 2: Overcome Fears

Susan Jeffers is a bestselling author, self-help guru, and motivational speaker. In her book *Feel the Fear and Do It Anyway*, she compares the alternatives of failing to a lack of action. In her assessment, not taking action is exponentially more damaging than failure. Lack of action in the face of fears leads to incomplete and unfulfilled experiences and accomplishments, perhaps the greatest tragedy of all. People of success and happiness, she argues, muster the strength to face their doubts head on and take action in the face of them.

Franklin D. Roosevelt once said, "The only thing we have to fear is fear itself." Whether it is fear of failure, abandonment, public speaking, or heights, the resulting non-action is most destructive. Alternatively, overcoming our fears is among the most exhilarating and empowering experiences we can ever have. Many of our students have a fear of public speaking. It is easy to understand how the inability to get up and communicate thoughts can limit one's future. People who fear abandonment are unable to enter into meaningful and positive relationships. We must recognize the destructive nature of our fears and seek to overcome short-term discomfort for the sake of the long-term realization of our dreams.

Step 3: Remove Limiting Beliefs

Have you ever felt like twenty-four hours is not enough time to accomplish everything you need to get done in a day? We are all very busy people. Whether you're raising a family, running a business, going to school, working one or more jobs, or all of the above, time is a precious commodity. We have kids who are very active in school, after school, and on the weekends. We run a large and growing global education company. We founded the Magic Wand Foundation, a non-profit organization dedicated to empowering youth. We go to the gym, stay involved in the community, walk our dogs, take our wives on dates, and find the time to read and try to improve ourselves. It's easy for us to run out of time and feel like there aren't enough hours in the day to do it all and do it well. But we've studied the ultra successful and determined that each one of them also had the same 24-hour days and 365-day years that we have. A lack of time is simply an excuse we make to rationalize the feeling that we're coming up short.

Dr. Wayne Dyer was one of the most notable bestselling authors and personal coaches in the world. In his book *Excuses Begone*, he discussed the limiting effect excuses have in our lives. Excuses, like fears, give us a reason to not do something, and when we do nothing, we all know what the results are. Some excuses might include "people can't change," "my situation is special," or "I'll do it tomorrow." As you can see, all of these prevent us from taking action; and new and purposeful action is the only way to alter our current path.

In addition to limiting beliefs, we all have thoughts that drain our energy and take us off our game. Anger, jealousy, and self-doubt are only a few of the emotions that divert our focus from what's really important in our lives. While it's unrealistic to remove all negative thoughts and emotions, it is critical that we learn to manage them and gain a higher level of control so we can maximize our potential. The *Sedona Method*, authored by Hale Dwoskins, is a powerful process that focuses on taking greater control of your thinking and channeling it toward more constructive things. NLP, or neurolinguistic programming, is another excellent approach to begin taking control of your limiting thoughts and beliefs. Do whatever works for you to start putting excuses in your rearview mirror.

Step 4: Accept Ownership of Your Results

John Wooden is considered one of the greatest coaches ever to coach any sport. He was named Coach of the Year six times. His UCLA Bruins Basketball team won ten national championships over a twelve-year period, including seven years in a row, and had a long-standing record of eighty-eight straight victories. Bill Walton, their remarkable center, once recounted an episode when UCLA was handed a rare loss. As the team went into the locker room, the finger of blame was being pointed in many different directions. The coaches had a bad game plan, the guards had too many turnovers, and the big men got out-rebounded. The team was divided, and Wooden saw an important opportunity. He stood up and took complete blame for the loss. He got out-coached and a simple adjustment he didn't make would have meant victory rather than defeat. As the team took a breath, finally not worrying about taking the blame for the defeat,

Wooden worked his magic. He pointed at Walton and asked him to explain what he could have done differently that would have changed the outcome of the game. Walton struggled for a minute, then came up with something that could have enabled victory. Each player who had played in the game proceeded to do the same, identifying how the loss was his fault.

As the locker room grew quiet, Wooden said, "Now we can all start the process of getting better." It was an epiphany for the players. They instantly realized that each of them was to blame, that every one of them could have done things differently that could have changed the outcome. That was something they could work on, something they could move forward with. Now the team was back to the process of getting better and controlling the outcome of their lives. UCLA went on to win the national championship again that year.

John Wooden epitomizes the *100% Accountable* Mindset, a recognition that you completely control everything that happens in your life. You are not a victim of your past, and your future has not been determined. You are what you decide you will be from this point and each moment going forward. You are the product of the decisions you make and the actions you take.

One other important aspect of this mindset is *Entitlement vs. Empowerment*. The mental habit of *entitlement* is a byproduct of the victim mentality. It is a belief that someone or some group owes you something. As soon as you buy into this, you give away your power to produce and create results in your life, by making your success and happiness dependent on others. People who achieve success and enjoy extraordinary happiness and meaning refuse to allow anyone else to dictate the course of their lives.

Step 5: Change What You Control

In his book *The Success Principles*, Jack Canfield presents a classic formula for the attainment of results in one's life. The formula, Event + Response = Outcome (E + R = O), explains that life is a series of events or circumstances to which we respond in some way. The combination of these events and our responses determines the outcome or results of our lives.

The secret to changing the circumstances of your life lies in this simple formula. We have developed a new, slightly different model of the formula, which demonstrates the power you have to not only change the outcomes in your life, but also improve all future events and circumstances.

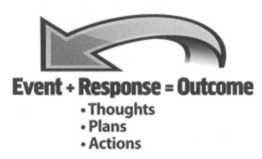

Event + Response = Outcome
- Thoughts
- Plans
- Actions

Our adjustment to the formula illustrates what we *do* control. These include the thoughts and emotions we have, the plans we make, and the actions we take. By adjusting these three elements, we can easily change the outcomes in our lives. Moreover, as we actively create more desirable outcomes in our lives, we begin to see a shift in the future events or circumstances of our lives. The result is a cycle of positive change, created simply by how we respond to the events we experience.

We can change the scope of our lives by changing the way we do things in the present. Every action we take has an equal and opposite reaction. If we change what we do, we change who we become.

An essential part of putting this life-changing formula into practice is measurement; not in the form of spreadsheets or statistical analysis, but rather by simply recognizing the positive shift. Like all people, we need positive feedback and affirmation that what we are doing is working. We must learn to recognize the little shifts. When we work out, we should pay attention to the improvement in our bodies. When we eat healthier, we should pay attention to the sensation of feeling better. If we adjust our management style, we must recognize how people are responding to us differently. The life changes we seek and the dreams we pursue are enabled by thousands of tiny steps. We must recognize the incremental improvements in our lives every step of the way.

Step 6: Become Truly Free

Viktor Frankl is one of the most extraordinary men of all time. In 1942, this respected psychologist, along with his new bride, mother, father, and brother were arrested by the Nazis in Vienna, Austria, and sent to concentration camps. Frankl spent three years living in some of the worst conditions known to modern man. When Dr. Frankl's concentration camp was liberated in 1945, he learned that his family had not survived.

What he observed in the extermination camp became the source of his "Logo Therapy." He noticed that those who lived had one thing in common: they had chosen to live rather than die. He found that when everything else had been taken—friends, food, dignity, and health— the one thing their captors could not take was choice … the choice to live. According to Frankl, the last of man's inalienable rights is the right of individuals to choose how they respond in any given situation. Frankl said, "Everything can be taken from a person but one thing, the last of human freedoms: to choose one's attitude in any set of circumstances, to choose one's own way."

Freedom is a word that has been passed down for generations. It is an idea linked to political or religious ideology. One definition of freedom is *a state in which someone is able to act and live as he or she chooses, without being subject to any undue restraint or restriction.*

We think of restraints or restrictions imposed on us as laws. What about the restrictions we place on ourselves? Every time we do something out of character that is influenced by someone else, we are in a form of bondage. We may act differently around friends, we may get nervous when people are watching, or we may not take action for fear of being rejected by someone else. Each of these is an example of giving away our freedom.

Frankl once said they could take everything away, they could strip him naked and starve him, but they would never get his pride, his thoughts, or his hope for the future. This is the essence of true freedom, unencumbered by the thoughts and opinions of others, in which our actions are intrinsic and of the greatest possible alignment with our dreams and who we are.

Mindset in a Minute

100% Accountable

Choose to be responsible for your own happiness and success.

Step 1. Reconcile with the past: Find a way to free yourself from issues in your past. Forgiveness begins and ends with you.

Step 2. Overcome fears: Recognize the destructive nature of your fears and take action, one step at a time, and you will start to experience the exhilaration of a breakthrough.

Step 3. Remove limiting beliefs: Realize that most limiting beliefs are self-imposed and have no basis in truth or validity. Try exchanging your limiting belief for the exact opposite positive thought.

Step 4. Accept ownership of your results: The process of self-improvement begins when you take complete ownership of your current situation. When you stand in the truth, you give yourself permission to grow.

Step 5. Change what you control: While you may not control all of the circumstances in your life, you do control how you react to them. Your thoughts, emotions and actions influence your future outcomes.

Step 6. Become truly free: Recognize that true freedom resides within you, and, regardless of circumstances, you control your own attitude. This is also a great reminder that you should not waste energy trying to control another person's life, but rather, allow that person the freedom of his own choices.

"If not now, when? If not here, where? If not me, who?"

–Steve Geiger

Attitude of Gratitude
Chapter 7

"If you change the way you look at things, the things you look at change."
—Wayne Dyer

Penny for Your Thoughts?

It's estimated that approximately 65,000 thoughts go through our minds every day. About ninety-five percent of these thoughts are the exact thoughts we had the day before and the day before that. What's on our minds basically stays on our minds. This wouldn't be so bad, except that about eighty percent of our thoughts are fueled by negativity. The term to describe this is *Automatic Negative Thoughts*, or ANTs. We are people of habit, so when the same negative thoughts repeat each day, we become conditioned to believe them, regardless of how pessimistic they are. Our brains keep serving us negative thoughts all day, every day; and for the majority of people, it hasn't been a fair fight … until now.

Bestselling author and leadership expert John Maxwell describes an interesting research study on professional athletes in his book, *Talent Is Never Enough*. According to Maxwell, professional athletes have twenty-five percent fewer thoughts each day than the average person. This by no means implies that they have fewer intellectual thoughts, just fewer negative thoughts. Their secret holds the key to positive change for the rest of us. It begins with the pros' understanding of how powerfully their thoughts affect their performance. Every day, they miss shots, throw interceptions, strike out, make bad plays and lose games. They don't want these negative memories to haunt them, so they use techniques to eliminate them and keep them from repeating every day. They simply have fewer negative thoughts, and it improves their performance. We will teach you some of these techniques so you can put them to work in your life.

It's fairly easy for most of us to be grateful for the good things in our lives. According to Martin Seligman's global research project on happiness, that's good news; because systematically being grateful can increase our lifespans. Seligman, the father of the positive psychology movement, has performed extensive studies on the impact of gratitude on our life experience. In one study, he tested people who were depressed. Each person was asked to spend a few minutes each day writing down the things for which they were grateful. The results were amazing. Ninety-two percent felt happier, ninety-four percent were less depressed, eighty-four percent felt less stressed, and seventy-eight percent had more energy. Even more amazing, the study estimated that by simply expressing daily gratitude, we can add 6.9 years to our lives—an impact superior to quitting smoking or performing regular exercise! Our research yielded several techniques for increasing gratitude in your daily life that we will share with you shortly.

However, there was one significant finding that we didn't expect.

An *Attitude of Gratitude* extends far beyond the typical things for which people tend to be thankful. In fact, the unexpected blueprint for an extraordinary life includes being grateful for your challenging situations too.

The Counter Mindsets

A study was performed in which people were asked about their experiences in the subway. Participants were asked what percentage of the time the train going in the opposite direction they were traveling arrived before the train they were waiting for. The overwhelming majority of travelers believed the other train came first more often. In fact, statistics showed that both trains came first fifty percent of the time. Termed the "Subway Fallacy," this study demonstrates a collective condition of our society. The anger and frustration created by the other train coming first created a more memorable experience. When the traveler's train came first, it created no indelible image or memory in the mind. People recall more of the negative experiences, hence the perception that the other train came more often. Unfortunately, we live in a world that is being conditioned more by negative experiences than positive ones.

In his book *Authentic Happiness*, Martin Seligman shares research which indicates that depression is ten times more prevalent today than it was in 1960. Unfortunately, it is also affecting much younger people: the average age has gone from 29.8 to 14.5 years old, and it has very little to do with money. Seligman's study shows that once household income reaches $8,000 per year per person, there is no correlation between any amount of money and happiness. As a matter of fact, real income in the U.S. has increased by sixteen percent over the last thirty years, while the number of people describing themselves as happy has decreased from thirty-six to twenty-nine percent.

Somehow, in the fast-paced world of today, we've lost sight of what matters most; we are no longer connected to the things that build meaning and happiness in our lives. The more we get, the more we focus on what we don't have; and with our energy focused on what we don't have, we're constantly seeking more and more. The following Mindset in Action steps will help you incorporate the *Attitude of Gratitude* Mindset into your daily life.

Mindset in Action: A Step-by-Step Approach

Step 1: Focus on the Positives

Martin Seligman believes that more than ninety-eight percent of psychologists make their money focusing on problems. His movement went against the grain, seeking ways to build from a foundation of positivity so that our children could become immune to many of the social and emotional problems we face today. There is a quote that says, "Energy flows where attention goes." What we focus our attention on is what expands in our life. Many people focus their attention on what they don't have, or on what they have and don't want. As long as their minds are focused on this lack, these challenges will persist and likely expand in their lives. Seligman is begging us to use positives as the foundation of our lives.

A common practice used by marriage counselors epitomizes the "focus on the positives" mentality. Typically, what happens in struggling marriages is a focus on what isn't working and each other's character flaws or personality deficiencies. When the attention goes to the negatives, that is where the energy of the relationship flows. Experts like Denis Waitley, Wayne Dyer, and Deepak Chopra describe a simple strategy that's been used by psychologists for many years. Simply stated, psychologists ask couples to write down all the things they like about the other person, and then instruct them to focus more and more on those things. What often happens next transforms marriages. The two begin seeing each other in a different light and more often find themselves in situations where the other is in his or her element. Both of their demeanors change, and a new positive energy comes to inhabit the relationship. By adjusting the focus of their attention, they begin enjoying far more positive results and feelings in their relationship.

When your mind is focused on scarcity and lack, it is impossible to begin leveraging your assets to build the life of your dreams. We have two choices in life: we can elect to focus on the negatives, or we can choose to build on all the positive things. If you choose the negatives, you risk living in a downward spiral. If you build from the positives, there is nowhere to go but up.

Step 2: Journal Your Gratitude

Oprah Winfrey is well known to keep a daily gratitude journal, a practice she was taught by her mentor, Maya Angelou. As Oprah put it:

> "I live in the space of thankfulness, and I have been rewarded a million times over for it. I started out giving thanks for small things, and the more thankful I became, the more my bounty increased. That's because what you focus on expands, and when you focus on the goodness in your life, you create more of it. Opportunities, relationships, even money flowed my way when I learned to be grateful no matter what happened

in my life."

The *Attitude of Gratitude* is not a one-time project, nor is it a series of incremental steps. It is a way of life that infuses energy into every aspect of your being. Napoleon Hill coined it *PMA*, or *Positive Mental Attitude*. It was the defining characteristic of people like Walt Disney, Dale Carnegie, and Norman Vincent Peale. Simply stated, a PMA causes you to expect more from each moment, and because of this, you extract more out of your time.

We suggest you keep a daily gratitude journal. In your journal, write down the obvious things for which you are grateful. This might include your health, family, and friends. Also include often-overlooked items such as the air you breathe, the water you drink, or even a beautiful flower. As Martin Seligman pointed out, keeping a daily journal of that for which you're grateful can even increase your lifespan. To really boost gratitude in your life, we would also suggest that you pay attention to the good things that happen to you each day, simply making a mental note of each event in your mind. Our research demonstrates that, at a minimum, you will feel happier with what you have, which can make all the difference in the world.

Step 3: Defuse the Negatives

Have you ever had one of those days that starts off wrong and seems to get worse and worse? Perhaps you oversleep and then stub your toe on the way to the bathroom. Maybe some toothpaste gets on your shirt and you have to change your clothes. Throughout the day, one misstep feeds into another. It doesn't take long for you to start stringing together one bad day after another, and then one bad week becomes a bad month and so on. This doesn't mean that everything that happens is bad, but it starts to feel like you might be in a rut. You may even feel like you're a magnet for misfortune. If you've ever felt like this, don't worry, because you aren't alone. Here's a technique you can use to defuse the negatives before they pile up. It's based on a process Scott developed and has taught to thousands of students. He explains:

> When I was a little boy, I was afraid of the dark. I needed a night light just to help me go to sleep. To this day, when I walk into a dark room I feel a bit uneasy. As soon as I flip the switch and the lights come on, I feel much better. Just like I walk into a dark room and turn on the light switch, I've learned to flip my emotional switch from negative to positive. I imagine I have an invisible light switch on my chest right on top of my heart. When I feel uneasy because a negative thought or emotion enters my stream of consciousness (one of those daily ANTs), I pretend to flip my imaginary switch from negative to positive. Basically, when I flip the switch, I stop giving any thought or emotion to what I don't want and replace what I'm thinking and feeling with something positive. Sometimes it's the exact opposite thought, and sometimes it's a completely different thought, as long as it's one that is purely positive.

Step 4: Thank It Forward

Do you remember the movie *Pay It Forward*? It came out in 2000, and the concept was so innovative that a national foundation called the Pay It Forward Foundation was created. The idea is that you can change the world by doing a favor for a few people with no expectation of being paid back. Instead, you ask those people to kindly pay it forward by doing three random favors for other people. Exponentially, these random acts of kindness can change the world for the better. Random acts of kindness are a great way to increase the level of gratitude you experience. It just feels great to do something nice for someone else with no expectation of anything in return. Our research demonstrated that the ultra successful believe that when they do a good deed, it comes back to them many times over.

Here's one more technique you might want to try. This was developed by one of our good friends, Christopher Koke. He suggests you seek out people to say thank you to each day. Saying thank you and meaning it is free and, therefore, not in limited supply. Often, the people closest to us, our family and friends, hear it the least. It's socially expected to thank our customers, vendors, and even colleagues for the obvious. Chris is suggesting something much deeper. He's talking about saying thank you on a really personal level.

Be on the hunt for things for which you can be thankful, and this will help redirect you from the typical list of things you wish would change. By focusing on gratitude and giving thanks, you will soon find that you have even more for which to be grateful. Chris also suggests, for a truly energizing experience, to consider adding a hug when appropriate. When you openly express thanks, you physically feel great. When another person receives an authentic thank you, they also feel good. This one is a real win-win.

Step 5: See Both Sides of the Coin

Scott says:

> *Every now and then I have a silly argument with my wife over the temperature in our house. I say, "It's hot in here," and she says, "It's cold." I walk over to the thermostat to prove my point. I read it aloud and tell her it's seventy degrees. Her*

reply is, "That's exactly what I said, it's cold in here." Then we argue whether seventy degrees is hot or cold. It's so silly, but we both tend to get worked up over it. After twenty years of marriage, these are not our best moments. Is it hot or is it cold? The answer is ... it just is. It's just seventy degrees. In this case, seventy degrees represents two sides of a coin. For me, it's hot, and for my wife, it's cold.

While this may seem like an insignificant thing to bring up, our research shows us that happy people tend to argue less often. They find ways to get along with others. They seek peaceful resolutions, and one way they accomplish this is by appreciating and accepting that other people have their own perspectives. As Dr. Phil McGraw, bestselling author of *Life Strategies,* says, "Even a flattened pancake has two sides." Learn to appreciate and acknowledge the views of others without having to prove your perspective as "right," and you will significantly increase your happiness factor.

Step 6: Become an Inverse Paranoid

Tony Robbins has successfully coached millions of people, including a number of presidents. He often describes the time in his life when his father left him and his family: One Thanksgiving, a man came to the door offering Tony's family some food. Tony's father was jobless, and the family was struggling. Tony's father was ashamed and became very angry, demanding the man leave and never come back. Later that night, Tony's father walked out the door and abandoned his family forever. At the time, it was the worst day of Tony's life.

As Robbins looks back on that day when a stranger made a charitable gift of food, he realized that it was the first time he understood that other people really did care about him and his family. When Tony was a bit older and his family was finally out of poverty's grip, he began giving away food every Thanksgiving. He would put the food by the door, ring the doorbell, and run away. He says those are some of the most powerful experiences of his life. Today, Tony has a foundation that feeds millions of people every year during Thanksgiving and Christmas.

On reflection, Tony considers the day his father left to be among the best days of his life. Instead of living a life fueled by emptiness, he started living a life filled with gratitude. The new gratitude he felt came from understanding that he was part of an amazing family of people whose lives are so full of joy and happiness that it flows out from them and into the lives of others, filling them like empty vessels. Once those vessels are full, they overflow, and the cycle of gratitude continues.

The term *Inverse Paranoid* was coined by W. Clement Stone, a businessman and philanthropist. The essential meaning of the term was handed down to people like Jack Canfield and Mark Victor Hansen of *Chicken Soup for the Soul* fame. Keep in mind, classic paranoia is described as the belief that the world and all in it are out to get you. Inverse Paranoids, on the other hand, truly believe some invisible force is constantly working for them, and not against them. They are vigilant in taking the good from all situations and using it to build toward their ultimate success.

We often asked the people we interviewed about defining moments in their lives—the time or occurrence they believed was the catalyst to their success. Invariably, they mentioned times of true adversity and challenge, and pointed to character traits that were developed or knowledge that was gained. If you talk to successful people, they will always point to the moments of adversity in their lives as the catalysts for their accomplishments. It is in the times of substantial challenge that character is built, knowledge is attained, and creativity is heightened.

Likewise, consider the things in your life that may not seem so positive. Become an Inverse Paranoid, and identify how those things will ultimately benefit you, possibly by teaching you a lesson or giving you a new perspective. When you experience challenging situations in life, especially serious tragedies, it's only human to feel loss, sorrow and even suffering. We hope you can find solace in the fact that it will only be a matter of time before you can look back with a greater sense of clarity on the situation. Perhaps your worst day will somehow become your best day.

"Keep your face to the sunshine, and you cannot see a shadow."

–Helen Keller

Mindset in a Minute

Attitude of Gratitude

Seek the positives from every experience, and be thankful for all you have.

Step 1. Focus on the positives: Remember the saying "energy flows where attention goes," focus on the positives, and make them the foundation upon which to build everything else in your life.

Step 2. Journal your gratitude: Constantly recognize the good things that happen in your life. Pay attention to and record the positive things that happen to you each day.

Step 3. Defuse the negatives: Learn to dismiss the ANT's (automatic negative thoughts) by flipping the switch from negative thoughts and emotions to positive ones.

Step 4. Thank it forward: Make time to thank people in your life for big and small things, and look to perform random acts of kindness.

Step 5. See both sides of the coin: Understand that each person has his own unique perspective, and learn to accept and appreciate that opinion without having to prove yourself right. Work hard not to judge things as good or bad, right or wrong. Accept everything that happens as a wonderful, natural unfolding of your life and dreams.

Step 6. Become an Inverse Paranoid: Like the most successful people, learn to expect that good things will happen to you. Assume the universe is conspiring to do you good, and even when things feel negative, believe that good will come of them and seek it out.

"Life is not about waiting for the storms to pass ... it's about learning how to dance in the rain."

–Vivian Greene

Live to Give
Chapter 8

"We make a living by what we get, but we make a life by what we give."
—Winston Churchill

A Social Adventure

People who live lives of achievement and happiness get more out of life because they give more. The vast majority of society believes in one of two paths: Either you achieve a certain level of financial means and then start giving to charity, or you give first, sowing the seeds along your journey. Our research found many examples of people in both categories, just as we anticipated. What we didn't expect was a much deeper meaning and execution of what we call the *Live to Give* Mindset. For starters, the concept of giving, in the world of the ultra successful, is most accurately defined as giving your best life to the world. In other words, being the best *you* possible. In their bestselling book *The Go-Givers*, authors Bob Burg and John David Mann describe this principle as "The Law of Authenticity," stating, "The most valuable gift you have to offer is yourself."

Interestingly, the way the people we researched have been able to live their best lives is by thoroughly embracing the *Passion First* Mindset. Because they are aligned with their authentic passions and strengths, they execute their lives better; they accomplish more, and consequently give more to the world around them. Quite simply, they create more value.

We create value in this world when we do things that are positive and constructive. When we create value, we have an impact. When our actions are positive and purposeful, the impact we have on ourselves and on others is beneficial. The beauty of the *Live to Give* Mindset is that we get what we give. Science teaches us that every action triggers a reaction, and that the energy we give off never dies, it only changes forms. When we create positive value in the world, the world responds in kind. We are usually compensated in the form of monetary income, but often the currency that has greater value is psychic income or a feeling of significance. When we live to our best, striving toward our fullest potential, we feel a greater sense of worth, accomplishment, and positive impact. This alone increases our sense of happiness, joy and fulfillment. It would almost appear to be selfish if it were not for the amazing side effects. When we give all that we can possibly give, the world is a better place.

Consider Martin Luther King, Jr., endowed with tremendous charisma and the ability to inspire, who aligned his abilities around the causes of equality and fighting segregation. The alignment of his unique abilities within the context of his life propelled him to a life of meaning and afforded him the opportunity to make extraordinary contributions to the world. The same can be said of Mother Teresa, Nelson Mandela, and Mahatma Gandhi. Lives of great meaning are led from an orientation toward service and the sharing of oneself to the advantage of others.

There is one final observation that seems to be a game changer in the land of extraordinary living. When people connect their passions to causes they believe in, the multiplier effect on their contributions to society is off the charts. We're not talking about surface giving, like when businesses donate a small percentage of their profits to charity. We're not knocking that by any means, but there seems to be an entirely different level of living to give when businesses are built around doing well while doing good.

The late Anita Roddick was one of our interview subjects who clearly fit this description. At thirty-three years old, Roddick was a housewife who opened a store in Brighton, England, to support herself and her two children. She barely had enough money for the rent. What she did have was a passion for environmentally friendly products, fair trade, and a host of other social causes she actively and openly supported through in-store signs and significant donations. She was a leader in social responsibility before most people even knew what that meant. She turned the tables on social responsibility and made it into more of a social adventure as she grew her tiny store, The Body Shop, into more than 1,000 retail locations in over 40 countries. Wanting to make the point that anyone, from practically any means, can make a difference, Anita shared this off-the-cuff quote: "If you think you're too small to have an impact, try going to bed with a mosquito in the room."

The Counter Mindsets

Does charity begin at home? Can we only give our money and time when we have more of both? Is our work about making a living?

These are very rational and practical questions. Is it possible that saving our good graces for ourselves and our families is limiting our lives? Could it be possible that the best way to earn more money and time is to give them both first? These may seem like counterintuitive concepts, but our research demonstrates that the ultra successful seem to experience a different reality.

In his book *The 7 Spiritual Laws of Success*, Deepak Chopra says that the universe has a perfect accounting system. His point is simply that we get out of life exactly what we give, every single time. Most of us live in a world imprisoned by the perception of scarcity. We must get *ours* because there is not enough to go around. We often ask, "What's in it for me?" It is this mentality that cuts off the flow of abundance in our lives. We shut off connections to so many new opportunities that come through the process of giving and sharing of ourselves. We drastically limit the value we create, which in turn decreases the value we receive.

We get paid for the work we do, yet many of us are left wanting more. You get out of relationships what you put into them, yet most of us seek deeper meaning and connections. We are what we eat, yet most people desire greater health and wellness. Everything we are and ever will be is a product of the things we do to attain them. We must do more to get more, because the universe may truly have a perfect accounting system.

And what about the work we do? We must re-orient how we perceive that as well. Today, one of the strongest measures of job quality is salary. Most of us seek employment with the hope of getting the highest financial return for the work we do. As discussed in the *Passion First* chapter, this can ultimately act in direct opposition to success, happiness, and even financial return. We must seek employment that provides us the greatest opportunity to serve, create value, and maximize our positive impact. When we do this, we create more value, and as a result, more value is showered upon us. Giving of our time, talent, and treasure does not need to feel like a responsibility, but rather an opportunity with an incredible return on investment: an extraordinary life!

Mindset in Action: A Step-by-Step Approach

Step 1: Share Your Unique Genius

Nature teaches us many lessons, but none as profound as the true essence of service. Consider an oak tree. The best thing an oak tree can do is grow to its fullest potential. The larger its size, the more shade it provides, the more leaves it drops that nourish the soil, the more acorns to feed the animals, and the more life-giving oxygen it produces for the surrounding habitat. The seemingly selfish act of feeding itself with sunlight and soil nutrients empowers the oak to do the most good, not only for itself, but also for the world around it.

Bill Gates has donated billions of dollars to charity. All of this money is going toward wonderful causes that are benefitting millions if not billions of people. However, no amount of money donated by Gates will equal the impact Gates has had through the creation of Microsoft, and the software revolution he helped drive. Oprah, like Gates, is a generous philanthropist. That being said, the impact Oprah has had on improving the lives of millions of people through her talk show and other media outlets will never be equaled through her charitable giving.

The greatest contribution any of us can ever make for our family, community, and the world is simply to achieve our maximum potential. When we find our unique genius and align it with the world around us, we maximize our positive impact. We accomplish more, and we ultimately get more in return.

Step 2: Give Before You Get

Blake Mycoskie is an entrepreneur and the founder of TOMS Shoes. In 1996, he took a trip to Argentina, where he became interested in a rope-soled shoe that Argentinean farmers had been wearing for over a hundred years. Not only did Blake notice these unusual shoes, he also couldn't help but notice how many people, mostly children, were shoeless. He learned that because so many people couldn't afford shoes, they had no choice but to go barefoot. Being shoeless increased their risk of life-threatening diseases caused by bacteria in the soil entering the body through cuts and scrapes on the feet. Around the world, more than 300 million children are shoeless. Over one million children die each year from preventable diseases, simply because they have no shoes. Millions more don't attend school because they can't meet the basic dress code or sustain the journey to travel to school without footwear.

TOMS shoes was created with a new business model based on a one-for-one principle. For every pair of shoes TOMS sells, one pair is donated to a child in need. After selling 10,000 pairs of shoes from his apartment, Blake returned to Argentina with friends, loved ones, and his new TOMS family to hand-deliver 10,000 pairs of shoes to kids in need. Following his success in Argentina, Blake went to South Africa, where he hand-delivered 50,000 pairs of shoes to children. Since its founding, TOMS has donated more than 1 million pairs of shoes to children around the world. Recently, TOMS introduced a new product, sunglasses, with the same one-for-one model. For every pair of sunglasses sold, they provide sight-giving cataract surgery to someone in need.

When Napoleon Hill studied the most successful men and women in the history of the United States, he found a number of unifying qualities that separated them from the masses. In *Think and Grow Rich,* he stated that one of those qualities was, "They give before they get." In other words, the best way to start the flow of abundance in your life is to begin the process of giving and serving others. Blake has been able to grow his for-profit business faster than most shoe companies, in spite of the fact that he has no advertising budget. The initial advice he received from consultants was to first establish a financially sound business, and then begin donating shoes. While this made rational sense, Blake opted to give first and right from the very beginning.

Step 3: Seek Ways to Serve

Harris Rosen grew up in the Lower Eastside of New York City. His family was poor and barely scraped by. Harris learned to swim at the local Boys' Club, which provided programs and services to city kids in need. Nearly sixty years later, he still swims every day— only now he swims at one of the seven hotels he owns in Orlando, Florida. When we interviewed Harris, he spoke of how important it is to serve others. He mentioned that anyone could do it simply by being friendly and generous with his or her time. He reflects fondly on his days at the Boys' Club, citing that it was less about a place to swim and more about connecting with caring individuals who were genuinely concerned for his well-being. Today, Harris employs over

4,500 people and has his own staff of doctors and nurses that provides onsite medical benefits for employees and their families. Perhaps this is the reason why he has one of the highest retention rates in the hospitality industry in his area. He also thinks it's one of the reasons his team goes out of their way when serving guests at any of the Rosen Hotels & Resorts. Service is contagious and, remarkably, both the giver and receiver feel a sense of empowerment.

Mr. Rosen is an amazing entrepreneur who lives the *7 Mindsets*. We learned why *Forbes* magazine named him one of the most generous philanthropists in America. Harris has adopted the disadvantaged community of Tangelo Park in Florida. He provides free pre-school for all of the two-, three-, and four-year-old children from the neighborhood. He also makes a promise to every young person from the community that if he or she graduates from high school and is accepted into a vocational school, community college, or four-year public university in Florida, he will pay the full tuition, room and board. To date, he has provided hundreds of scholarships and has plans to continue inspiring local students to reach new heights.

Each of us has opportunities to serve others every day, whether at work, at home, in school, or around the community. It begins with having a generous heart and recognizing that even the little things make a big difference. Lao Tzu once said, "He who gathers has little, and he who scatters has much." The irony is that he who scatters gathers more. The best way to create abundance in your life is to start the cycle that begins with serving others.

Step 4: Align with Your Passions

Serving others can and should be one of the most inspiring and engaging activities in which we participate. We like to call it the social adventure of our lives. To live up to the motto, we must align who and what we serve with the activities and causes that matter to us. When we do this, it becomes highly relevant, it becomes exciting, and the objectives of the effort become critically important to us as individuals. As you might imagine, our chances of having more success and heightened meaning increase exponentially. Thus, we gain more meaning and are much more likely to perform similar activities in the future.

If we look at philanthropists and achievers, their success is predicated on a cause that is of fundamental importance to them. For Mother Teresa, it was serving the impoverished people of India. For Gandhi, it was freeing the oppressed. And for Martin Luther King, Jr., it was ending segregation. It was the purpose that created the passion that drove the activity that accomplished the goal.

Look for ways to incorporate authentic giving in all you do. Connect your passion with a purpose larger than yourself. Whether through a business, a job, or volunteer work, aligning your passion with a *Live to Give* Mindset will increase your sense of purpose, happiness, and positive impact on others.

"Do all the good you can, by all the means you can, in all the ways you can, in all the places you can, at all the times you can, to all the people you can, as long as ever you can."

–John Wesley

Mindset in a Minute

Live to Give

Inspire and serve others while you maximize your potential.

Step 1. Share your unique genius: Understand that the greatest contribution any of us can make is to leverage our unique talents, strengths, and passions and share them with the world to the maximum extent possible.

Step 2. Give before you get: Know that the best way to get what you want in life is to give first. Once you start creating value for others, the world responds in kind with greater abundance in your life.

Step 3. Seek ways to serve: Incorporate the mentality of service in every aspect of your life. Understand the value of your life is the sum of the impacts you have. Seek to have the greatest possible positive impact in everything you do.

Step 4. Align with your passions: Make the benefits of what you do be of profound importance to who you are and the legacy you want to leave with your life. When you do this, you will invigorate everything you do, create greater value with your actions, and ultimately receive greater benefit in return.

"A candle loses nothing by lighting another candle."

–Father James Keller

The Time Is Now
Chapter 9

"It is not the critic who counts; not the man who points out how the strong man stumbles, or where the doer of deeds could have done them better. The credit belongs to the man who is actually in the arena, whose face is marred by dust and sweat and blood, who strives valiantly, who errs and comes up short again and again, because there is no effort without error and shortcoming, but who does actually strive to do the deeds, who knows great enthusiasms and great devotions, who spends himself for a worthy cause; who at the best knows in the end the triumph of high achievement, and who at the worst, if he fails, at least fails while daring greatly, so that his place shall never be with those cold and timid souls who neither know victory nor defeat."

–President Theodore Roosevelt

An International Hero

Fred DeLuca is the founder of SUBWAY®, arguably one of the most successful restaurant franchises in the world. We interviewed Fred and discussed his book, *Start Small, Finish Big*, to get his perspective on the nature of living big dreams. In his words, "You simply have to start by taking small steps." Subway is a classic example of a young man taking small but purposeful steps. Many of DeLuca's early actions were ill-fated. On the opening day of his first restaurant, he only had one knife to cut the sandwiches. He wasn't prepared, the line of people became frustrated, and many left.

His first store didn't make a profit, and he thought about closing the business. He was conflicted, because he had a goal to open five sandwich shops within five years. He knew that if he closed this store, even if it was losing money, he would be moving in the opposite direction of his goal. Against the advice of others, he opened a second store, which also lost money. It took five years, five stores, and a significant amount of struggle before his concept started to work. Success for DeLuca came with time because he acted, he learned, and he adjusted. This is the process of success. Rarely does someone achieve greatness because of one magnificent moment. On the contrary, success is comprised of a thousand tiny but meaningful steps that ultimately result in dream realization. As Fred puts it, "Starting small is better than never starting at all."

"To achieve greatness, start where you are, use what you have, and do what you can."

–Arthur Ashe

The Time Is Now Mindset delivers the power to activate your Ultimate Life and enjoy the journey every step of the way. Learning the 7 Mindsets and living them are two completely different things. You've probably heard the saying, "Knowledge is power," but it's the implementation of the knowledge that leads to the power. This isn't necessarily a revelation, but there does seem to be a significant difference in the level of action between the ultra successful and the average person. In our interview with Mark Victor Hansen, co-author of the *Chicken Soup for the Soul* series, he pointed out the huge gap between what people know and what they do. In this chapter, we will share our research-based findings on what you can do now to activate the Mindsets in your daily life.

The Counter Mindsets

"Good things come to those who wait." As well-intentioned as this saying may be, it has the potential to completely derail your dreams. So many people fail to reach their potential because they simply don't take enough action. Perhaps they hesitate because they are unsure of the path to take. Maybe it's fear that holds them back. Or it could be that they are waiting for others to join them or lead the way. What we do know is that far too many people end up settling in life, when the difference between ordinary and extraordinary can literally be one extra step in the direction of their dreams.

There are two other memes we believe contribute to inactivity. We want to point these out, because freeing yourself from their grip can make all the difference. Growing up, we all became familiar with the saying, "Don't make the same mistake twice." When parents say this, their intent is to teach children to learn from their mistakes and make the necessary adjustments to get it right the next time. When we ask students what this means to them, they tell us it has taught them that mistakes are bad. Unfortunately, that is a huge disconnect and does a great deal of harm.

How about the warning, "If it ain't broke, don't fix it"? Did you know that when Albert Einstein was a young man, many physicists believed that they knew everything there was to know about the workings of the universe? From their perspective, it wasn't "broken." Luckily for us, Einstein didn't believe what other physicists believed, because he developed his theory of relativity and changed everything; as a result, the world is now a much different place.

We have conditioned acceptance into our culture. We are teaching ourselves not to challenge the status quo; and worse, we are not acting on our dreams and inspirations. Newton's law of motion says that every action has an equal and opposite reaction. Failure to act manifests into a failure to get results. Learn to embrace *The Time Is Now* Mindset, and you will experience a new world of possibilities.

"Take the first step in faith. You don't have to see the whole staircase, just take the first step."

–Dr. Martin Luther King, Jr.

Mindset in Action: A Step-by-Step Approach

Step 1: Enjoy Now

Eckhart Tolle is the bestselling author of *The Power of Now* and *The New Earth*. In his books, Tolle focuses on the concept of "presence," which simply translates into the ability to stay completely in the current moment. Our ability to do this galvanizes our effectiveness as individuals and increases the depth of meaning in our lives. Tolle would certainly agree with the quote by Bill Keane, "Yesterday is history, tomorrow is a mystery, but today is a gift ... and that is why they call it the present."

Somehow, over the course of our lives, we have been desensitized to the amazing beauty and wonder that surround us. Claude Monet once said that if he could create the world on a blank canvas, he would be unable to create anything more beautiful and spectacular than what nature has created for us. From the colors of the rainbow, the air we take in, and the cool water we drink, life is truly a gift that we often take for granted.

If you think about it, the true measure of one's quality of life is the sum of the moments he or she spends on earth. Learn to find pleasure in the moment. Enjoy each and every moment as the singular and wonderful experience it is. Embrace the time and place you're in and the people you're with. To improve the quality of your life, find more meaning and joy in the now. Do this often enough, and you will begin stringing together more and more moments of peace and joy.

Step 2: Understand that Everything You Do Matters

The Butterfly Effect is a scientific concept based on the chaos theory. The namesake "Butterfly" comes from the notion that a butterfly flapping its wings in one part of the world could cause a hurricane on the other side. This scientific theory teaches us the incredibly interconnected nature of all things. It helps us understand how everything we do matters, not just to us, but to everyone and for all time.

Writer and speaker Andy Andrews expands on this concept when telling the story of Raymond Baker, who was given an award for hydrolyzing corn, a process credited with providing food for and saving over two billion lives in impoverished areas around the world. Andrews explains that Baker had been hired by Henry Wallace, Vice President of the United States under President Franklin D. Roosevelt, to run a lab to hydrolyze corn. Henry Wallace had been a protégé of George Washington Carver, who had instilled in Wallace a passion for agriculture and using his skills to solve major world issues. George

Washington Carver's life had been saved by a young farmer named John Bentley, a stranger hired by Moses Carver to find George, his mother and brother, all of whom had been kidnapped by a team of raiders. George's mother was sold into slavery, and he never saw her again. Moses Carver and his wife raised Carver and his brother as their own sons and provided them with a first class education, something unheard of in Carver's time.

Andrews' point is that while Baker was credited with saving two billion lives, untold actions had been taken by others throughout history that set the stage for Baker to hydrolyze corn and save those lives. If Bentley had not saved Carver's life and put him on the road to greatness, then perhaps Baker would have never saved two billion lives—an example of the Butterfly Effect in action. Sir Isaac Newton once said, "If I have seen farther than others, it is because I have stood on the shoulders of giants." Andrews emphasizes that our actions matter not only to us, but to everyone. Everything we do impacts our lives and sends ripples flowing outward forever. Nothing you do is insignificant.

Step 3: Get in the Zone

We once had the opportunity to hear the Dalai Lama speak in Atlanta. He was asked what he felt about the United States, and what he thought was our deepest need. He simply stated that he wished more of us would seek to act from a place of warm-heartedness. What the Dalai Lama calls warm-heartedness is simply an expression of good feeling. It can be love, gratitude, empathy, compassion, or joy. It is when we are at our best and when the things we do have the greatest possible impact on the world around us.

Success is predicated on our ability to act from a position of strength.

At the very core of this is how we feel at the time we perform the action. Parents know how much more effective they are when love or empathy is driving their actions versus anger and frustration. Deepak Chopra once gave this simple advice to parents: "Be only love, and show only love." His meaning is simple. If our actions are driven by love, whether they are stern words of discipline or kind words of recognition, those actions will be positive and in the best interests of the child.

Perhaps the greatest things any of us can do are learn to manage our emotions, understand when we are off our path, and rein in the negativity to avoid doing harm to ourselves and others. With practice, you can learn to flip the switch and alter your emotions so that you act from a position of strength. Athletes call this place the *zone*, a state of heightened and often optimal performance. This is not a condition that should be reserved for athletes, but one you should learn to incorporate into your life on a regular basis. When you're feeling stressed or angry, you are not in the zone. Try taking a deep breath, relax, and tune into the zone before taking important actions.

Step 4: Be a Continuous Learner

Michael Jordan took the game-winning shot fifty-one times during the course of his college and professional career—he missed twenty-six times. Babe Ruth is considered one of the greatest home run hitters, but he also led the league in strikeouts for 5 years, striking out 1,330 times! That's almost twice the number of home runs he hit. The Wright Brothers were ridiculed during many of their failed attempts at flight. The point is that some of the most famed accomplishments of all time have been riddled with failure, yet few people remember the failures—they remember the achievements.

We live in a world of cause and effect. To get a result, something must happen. That is simply a fact. To get results, we must act. We cannot get hung up on the past, and we can't afford to wait for everything to line up perfectly, because it never will. What often gets in the way is fear of failure and fear of the unknown. When we asked the ultra successful what their impression of risk was, the overwhelming majority rarely saw anything they ever did as risky. They simply took action with expected outcomes, and when the outcomes were not what they'd expected, it became a learning experience from which they could grow and get better. They seem to have a certain comfort with uncertainty, and they prepare themselves to adjust as they gather new data.

The fundamental ingredients to success are the constant initiative to take action in conjunction with the inherent mentality to continually learn and adjust from the experience. What most people call failure, successful people call feedback. Ambrose Redmond once said, "Courage is not the absence of fear, but the ability to act in the face of it." Genius, then, comes from understanding that failure occurs only when you don't learn from it.

Step 5: Act on Purpose

Beck Weathers was part of an ill-fated Mt. Everest expedition that took place in May of 1996. On that day, the climbers were caught at the top of the mountain in a terrible storm that left eight dead, including two of the most experienced high altitude climbers in the world. Weathers lost the use of his eyes due to the effects of the high altitude. Buried in the snow, he was left for dead by some other climbers who came upon him and believed him to have already died.

Jeff met Beck Weathers one evening when Weathers was giving a presentation in Atlanta. During his speech, he described being trapped in the snow and left for dead. Hours into the ordeal, he had a clear vision of his wife and children. Unable to fathom not being with them again, he simply found the energy to stand up. In an amazing display of intuition, he was able to traverse the mountain and find a group of tents, where he was cared for before being taken to safety.

Action is something we must take to keep our lives moving forward. And if we can infuse action with the passion of authentic purpose, the power of our action increases exponentially. Consider the high level of performance you see from Olympic athletes. Think of humanitarians such as Martin Luther King, Mother Teresa, and Mahatma Gandhi, whose actions were motivated by something that transcended their individual lives. Recall great heroes like Joan of Arc, Winston Churchill, and the millions of unnamed men and women who have performed incredible acts of bravery, all of whom were inspired and moved by a greater purpose. We must find our inspiration, and we must act on it. When we do, the power of our actions will take us much further down the pathway to an extraordinary life.

"Nobody can go back and start a new beginning, but anyone can start today and make a new ending."

—Marianne Williamson

Mindset in a Minute

The Time Is Now
Harness the power of this moment and take purposeful action today.

Step 1. Embrace the moment: Understand that the moment is all you have and, in many ways, the meaning of your life will be determined by how much joy you find in each one.

Step 2. Understand that everything you do matters: Per the Butterfly Effect, every action you take sends ripples throughout the world that go on forever. Know this, and seek to make all your actions positive and purposeful.

Step 3. Get in the zone: Put yourself in a position to perform at your optimal level. This means getting in a positive mood, quieting your mind, and becoming present in the moment before you take significant action.

Step 4. Be a continuous learner: Understand that in life there is no failure, only feedback. Get comfortable with uncertainty and prepare to adjust as you learn from your experiences.

Step 5. Act on purpose: When you know what you want from your life and what matters, seek to take more and more actions toward your dreams, and eliminate as many non-value-added activities from your life as possible.

The Time Is Now

The Man Who Thinks He Can

If you think you are beaten, you are;
If you think you dare not, you don't.
If you'd like to win, but think you can't,
It's almost a cinch that you won't.
If you think you'll lose, you're lost,
For out in the world we find
Success begins with a fellow's will;
It's all in the state of mind.

If you think you're outclassed, you are:
You've got to think high to rise.
You've got to be sure of yourself before
You can ever win a prize.
Life's battles don't always go
To the stronger or faster man;
But sooner or later the man who wins
Is the one who thinks he can.

–Walter D. Wintle

Live Your Dreams
Chapter 10

"All our dreams can come true if we have the courage to pursue them."
—Walt Disney

Let the Transformation Begin

Now you've learned the *7 Mindsets,* and it is time to start living them. Personal change can be very difficult. Earlier in the book, we stated that many experts believe over ninety-eight percent of self-improvement efforts fail. Bryan Tracy, bestselling author and world-renowned life coach, states that the greatest enemy of personal change is the power of suggestion. No matter how inspired you are to change, you have to execute the change in the same environment and influences that created the very habits you are trying to adjust. Over his long career, Tracy has learned that success is predicated on sustainability, which requires an empowerment model that becomes part of the power of suggestion and delivers information, motivation, and inspiration to help an individual adjust his or her mental habits and mindsets.

We have divided this chapter into two sections. The first contains a list of research-based suggestions and ideas to help you get started and, more importantly, sustain the positive changes you initiate. In section two, we provide an overview of the sustainability process we have tested with several thousand people over the past several years. Personal improvement is a very individual process. In the end, it is up to you and only you to define and execute this change within yourself. We have, however, identified a variety of critical elements that, when implemented, we believe will significantly improve your level of success.

Section One: Suggestions for Sustainability

Radical Self-Interest

To increase your chances of success, you have to be able to answer the personal question, "What's in it for me?" The results of your efforts must *matter* to you. This is where you'll get the initial motivation to start the process. Extreme examples of this are when people find out they have a serious medical issue and need to make a radical change to their lifestyle. When this is the case, they become highly motivated to make a change and stick with it. The stakes are high, and there is little room for error. This process is something that you can replicate for other changes you want to make in your life. The best way to light the fire is to envision the new life you desire and the benefits you'll reap from your improved effort. Visualizing what your life will look like and how you will feel after you've made the change will help put you in the proper frame of mind.

The Power of the Pack

While the process of change is personal, your chances of success are substantially improved with a collective effort. People who exercise almost always achieve better results when they have a partner or a group of people committed to inspiring and holding each other accountable. A great team is always stronger than the sum of its parts. The point is, any significant life change will require support from others along the way. Many people find increased inner strength and resilience when they help support others going through the same life-changing process as they are. Find a *Mindset Buddy*, or start your own Ultimate Life Club with friends, coworkers, or family; you'll experience the power of the pack—when two or more people committed to a common goal do whatever it takes to help each pack member achieve new levels of success.

Measure the Milestones

Most people want instant results and instant gratification when they implement a new approach. Experts agree that to lose weight and sustain it, you should lose approximately one pound a week. This seems too slow for most people, especially when they see an advertisement to lose ten pounds in ten days. While it's possible to lose more weight in a short period of time, the term yo-yo dieting exists because it's almost impossible to sustain weight lost in a rapid process. Know when going into any new routine that true and sustainable change happens slowly. Set small attainable goals that can be measured on a daily or weekly basis. It really is the little things that, when done over and over again, create the greatest long-term results. It's critical to recognize even the most marginal of milestones. This reinforces your resolve and builds confidence that you are getting where you want to go. Change comes through the execution of new and purposeful action that takes you places and creates new growth that did not exist before.

Expect the Unexpected

Everyone encounters roadblocks when they attempt to make changes in their lives. Sometimes, we can anticipate what they'll be, and other times we get completely surprised. There are major differences in how people react to the challenges that inevitably get in the way of success. Typically, those who push through the roadblocks and make positive changes are the ones who expected to hit a roadblock in the first place. They may not have known exactly what was coming, but were mentally prepared so that, when obstacles did materialize, they were prepared to adjust and find ways around them. Whatever the obstacles turn out to be, these people persevere and push forward. Those that typically fail to sustain their change have an entirely different reaction to setbacks and roadblocks. When something gets in their way and temporarily halts their progress, they view these things as proof that they can't make the changes needed, or that they knew it was going to be too hard. The obstacles become not just an excuse to stop, but a validation that the process for change is flawed. Our advice to you is to expect the unexpected and prepare to make changes, no matter what it takes and whenever it's needed. As Willie Jolley states in his book *It Only Takes a Minute to Change Your Life*, "A setback ain't nothin' but a setup for a comeback."

Section Two: The 7 Mindsets Experience

We have been teaching the *7 Mindsets* to tens of thousands of individuals, primarily teens and educators, for a number of years. We understand that real change gets measured over time, and that most people tend to forget what they learn unless they receive help to retain it.

Life is one of the best teachers, and our students need to experience situations over time that continually challenge what they're learning.

We developed and gradually improved a process and set of tools to help people deepen their understanding of the *7 Mindsets,* as well as activate and sustain them in their lives. We wanted to be there for them and also develop a process that could scale in order to reach and support millions globally. Internally, we call this Mindset Maintenance, a year-round process that engages and supports individuals in an ongoing way. The major components are:

Daily Inspiring Quotes (Morning Mindsets) – Every day, we distribute a quote that connects to one of the *7 Mindsets* via email and social media. Feedback indicates that these quotes help anchor the mindset concepts while also providing a continuous source of motivation and inspiration. Subscribe to the email version via our website (7Mindsets.com) or view the graphic versions via our social media profiles:

Facebook.com/7Mindsets	Twitter.com/7Mindsets
Pinterest.com/7Mindsets	Instagram.com/7Mindsets

Blog Posts – We distribute articles detailing ideas and techniques for how to positively leverage the *7 Mindsets.* Reference points often include little-known facts about famous and successful individuals, as well as unique personal experiences from *7 Mindsets* team members. These are posted on our website, 7Mindsets.com, and distributed via social media as well as through our email mailing list.

The *7 Mindsets* MasterClass – Our online training course for individuals delivers the *7 Mindsets* concepts through short, empowering videos filled with inspirational and unconventional advice. The MasterClass also includes an individualized Life Planning guide, through which MasterClass users are guided through a series of exercises to help them apply the mindsets in their own lives. Read more at 7Mindsets.com.

Stay in Touch! – Join our mailing list to be notified of new programs and resources! Email us today at info@7Mindsets.com.

Learning the 7 Mindsets Is Eye-Opening Living Them Is Life-Changing

This book was written to provide you with an understanding of the *7 Mindsets* and an overview of how to activate them in your life. Over the years, we've learned that sustaining this information requires ongoing effort. We encourage you to follow the advice and suggestions we've included; we are confident they'll help you use what you've learned to live the life of your dreams!

"You cannot hold a torch to light another's path without brightening your own."
–Rumi

Afterword

From increasing violence to global warming to persistent poverty, our world is facing many great challenges, and it's often difficult to see realistic solutions. In addition to such massive global issues, our communities and families are facing their own complexities as well. As Einstein said, "We can't solve our problems using the same type of thinking that created them." We believe the *7 Mindsets* blueprint represents the new thinking that's needed. Positive change is possible, and it will come from an often-overlooked place: the hearts and minds of our youth.

Our goal is nothing short of a global mindshift, a quantum leap forward in the way we think about ourselves, our world, and those who inhabit it with us. We often think of quantum leaps as massive events. The reality is that great shifts in our world can be the result of narrowly focused efforts. Imagine if all children learn the *7 Mindsets* as seamlessly as they learn their ABCs.

Through our process, students will move from learning the *7 Mindsets* to living them. We can teach parents, educators, and youth leaders to facilitate this learning, and through technology, we can empower and support youth globally. We think this can be accomplished in as little as thirty minutes a week.

Visualize a world in which young people identify their unique gifts and share them to their greatest ability. They will dream bigger, live more passionately, empower others, embrace accountability, appreciate life, give unconditionally, and act with purpose. We imagine this every day, and we've created a youth empowerment movement to bring it to fruition.

If you believe in our mission, join us!

- Live the *7 Mindsets* and be the best *you* possible!

- Share this book or recommend it to others. For every book purchased, we will donate one to a deserving student. Visit 7Mindsets.com to purchase.

- Amplify your understanding of *the 7 Mindsets* through our online courses. Email info@7mindsets.com for more information.

- Bring us to your community to keynote a conference, deliver a seminar, or collaborate on a youth empowerment project. Learn more at 7Mindsets.com or email info@7mindsets.com.

- Help bring the *7 Mindsets* to your local school or youth organization with a **7 Mindsets Academy** program. Email us for details at info@7mindsets.com.

- Engage with our daily Morning Mindset inspirational quotes and weekly blog posts. Email info@7mindsets.com for subscription info or follow us on social media:

Afterword

Facebook.com/7Mindsets   Twitter.com/7Mindsets

Pinterest.com/7Mindsets   Instagram.com/7Mindsets

When you live the *7 Mindsets,* you no longer need a magic wand to live your Ultimate Life—you *become* the wand, and you'll realize that you had the power all along.

Live Your Dreams,

Scott & Jeff

Bring the 7 Mindsets to Your Classroom and Community

"It's what you learn after you know it all that counts."

–John Wooden

7 Mindsets is a company that delivers programs based on years of extensive research on personal achievement, success and fulfillment, and more than 100 combined years working directly with hundreds of thousands of young people.

Through our work, we have learned that every young person possesses incredible potential. Our methodology allows them to uncover this potential, take pride in their uniqueness, and begin putting their skills and interests to work building better futures for themselves and the world around them. Our integrated mission is to empower youth globally, and it is at the core of everything we do.

We offer a variety of ways to help bring the *7 Mindsets* into your community, including in-school programs, live and virtual training workshops, and independent learning options and tools.

Feel free to review the various opportunities and contact us to discuss how we can help with your empowerment plans!

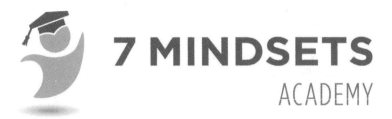

Empowering young people to pursue their best possible lives and helping prepare them for what lies ahead is both our privilege and passion. By shifting how they view the world and their place in it, the *7 Mindsets* help students experience a transformation that is immediate and permanent. Improved graduation rates, higher test scores, greater engagement, heightened character, and decreased behavior issues are all outcomes of learning the *7 Mindsets.*

7 Mindsets Academy is a social emotional learning program that changes the way students think, interact and live. Designed to easily assimilate into any school or youth organization's culture, 7 Mindsets Academy uses simple, powerful language to teach and activate success strategies, guiding students to avoid risk behaviors, pursue their dreams with a heightened sense of purpose, and feel empowered to make a meaningful difference in the world.

7 Mindsets Academy isn't about gaining more knowledge or new skills. Learning the *7 Mindsets* ignites a proactive, fundamental shift in a young person's character development that increases self-determination, academic performance, and resilience. With distinct curriculum levels for K-12, 7 Mindsets Academy programs can be implemented schoolwide or by individual classrooms in just minutes each week.

Contact us today if you'd like to learn more about bringing a 7 Mindsets Academy program to a school in your community!

7Mindsets.com

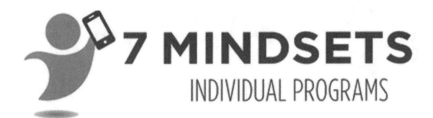

This book, *The 7 Mindsets to Live Your Ultimate Life*, represents the core of everything we've learned about the foundation of happiness and success. Available as an eBook, audiobook, and physical volume, it offers every individual who reads and shares it the opportunity to effect a phenomenal transformation in his or her own life and the lives of others.

To help maximize this opportunity, we have also developed a web-based personalized learning course to dramatically expand and deepen your understanding of the *7 Mindsets* from the convenience of any computer or device with Internet access.

The **7 Mindsets MasterClass** is an immersive learning experience that explores the actions and attitudes critical for a life of happiness and success. Presented as a series of online modules, the MasterClass utilizes research-based content, stories, videos, and an extensive life-planning process to connect what you learn with your dreams and desires. While learning the mindsets is eye-opening, living them is life-changing; and this program of engaging lessons and practical exercises is the key to building meaningful relationships, embracing the moment, acting with purpose, and learning how to live your ultimate life.

7Mindsets.com

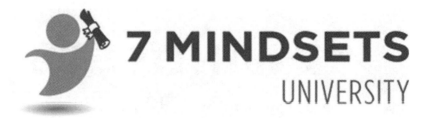

7 Mindsets University is a one-of-a-kind training experience in which attendees learn proven strategies for empowering students and educators to dream bigger, tap into their passions, work better with others, be more accountable and act with greater purpose.

A multi-day training event held at several locations across the country each year, 7 Mindsets University is delivered by dynamic youth empowerment leaders and world-class educators who are currently implementing the 7 Mindsets Academy social emotional learning program.

Get in touch to learn more about attending 7 Mindsets University, and begin positively changing lives forever!

7MindsetsUniversity.com

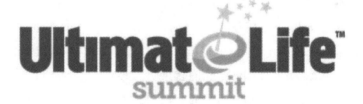

The **Ultimate Life Summit** (ULS) is a life-changing event that empowers young people with heightened optimism, unique life skills, and the thinking to begin living to their full potential. Much more than a summer camp, the Ultimate Life Summit is a truly unique experience.

Students from across the country and around the world convene for an immersive weeklong session to learn the *7 Mindsets* that lead to lives filled with passion, happiness, and extraordinary success. Conducted by some of the finest youth empowerment experts in the world, the ULS helps students identify their unique talents, raise their expectations for life, and learn to take daily action toward living their dreams.

Attendees take part in workshops and life-planning activities each morning and enjoy incredible fun attractions in the afternoon and evening, ensuring that the ULS is fast-paced, empowering, and filled with excitement from sunrise to sunset.

The ULS focuses on individual empowerment, self-determination, college and life planning, and leadership qualities to help attendees begin taking immediate action on their most important goals and dreams.

UltimateLifeSummit.com

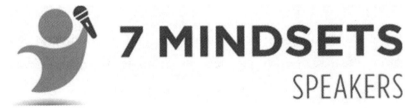

Bring the incredible power of the *7 Mindsets* to your organization, conference or community! Audiences will be captivated and supercharged with a new blueprint for happiness, meaning, and success through inspiring stories, powerful videos, and engaging activities.

From keynote presentations to multi-hour workshops for students, teachers, and corporations, our team will inspire and empower with the revolutionary thinking at the heart of happier, more successful lives!

7Mindsets.com

7 M*NDSETS

Teaching Mindsets. Changing Lives.

7 Mindsets offers proven products and programs for changing the way individuals think, interact and live, based on years of extensive research into the world's happiest and most successful people.

If you would like to help bring the *7 Mindsets* to schools, youth organizations, companies and individuals in your community while expanding your own business, consider becoming a *7 Mindsets* partner.

With a variety of approaches and program implementations available, the *7 Mindsets* partners program is a powerful way to augment your business objectives while helping spread the benefits of mindset education in your community or region.

If you're interested in empowering your community, contact us to discuss the *7 Mindsets* partner opportunity that's right for you!

Contact us at info@7mindsets.com.

About the Authors

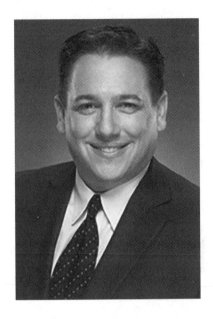

SCOTT SHICKLER is one of the world's leading experts on personal empowerment and entrepreneurship. *The Wall Street Journal* referred to him as "a serial and parallel entrepreneur" due to the number of businesses he has launched in diverse industries.

Collectively, Scott's companies have grossed over $100 million in business sectors from software to seminars and real estate to retail. He is the author or co-author of eight books, including *The Ultimate Entrepreneur* and *The 7 Mindsets to Live Your Ultimate Life*. Scott has been featured in a variety of media, including CNN, ABC and NBC News, *The New York Times* and *The Wall Street Journal*.

A graduate of Fordham University, Scott grew up in New York and now lives in Atlanta with his wife and two sons. In addition to his role with *7 Mindsets,* he is the co-founder of the Magic Wand Foundation, a non-profit organization devoted to empowering youth to live their dreams, as well as the founder of Excent Corporation, a global education software company serving millions throughout the world.

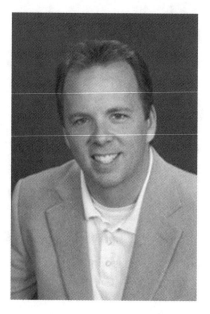

JEFF WALLER is a motivational speaker and thought leader on personal achievement and youth empowerment. He is the co-founder of Excent Corporation and the co-creator of 7 Mindsets, an organization focused on the delivery of cutting edge empowerment models distributed through scalable technologies on sustainable platforms.

Jeff is also the co-founder of the Magic Wand Foundation, an organization dedicated to empowering youth to make a positive impact on the world. His work includes the development of the revolutionary *7 Mindsets* program and the *Ultimate Life Summit,* a blended empowerment event that combines dynamic live seminars with existing and emerging tools to promote youth empowerment.

Jeff has dedicated the last decade to learning and understanding the critical elements that define high achievers. He has worked with thousands of teens, helping them identify their passions in life and encouraging them to pursue their dreams.

Prior to his work in youth empowerment, Jeff was a highly successful business strategist working with Fortune 500 companies. Jeff lives in Atlanta with his wife and three children. He holds a degree from The Georgia Institute of Technology.

Acknowledgements

"The future belongs to those who believe in the beauty of their dreams."
—Eleanor Roosevelt

This book is the culmination of our life's work—lives blessed with many extraordinary individuals along the way. We can only accomplish so much as individuals and, until we learn to work with, for, and through others, our big dreams will never be fulfilled. Along our journey, many individuals have taught us, coached us, and inspired us to be better and do better. All our dreams will forever be shared with those who have supported and inspired us along the way. It's virtually impossible to thank every person who has played a role in the research and writing of this book, but we do want to highlight some very special people:

Mitch Schlimer (Doc) – Mitch's experience and research has driven much of our thinking and methodology. More importantly, his friendship and guidance have brought us through many challenges and given us the strength and courage to pursue our destiny.

Juan Casimiro (Papi) – Juan has dedicated his life to helping youth.

He is an inspiration to all who know him and understand the depths of his empathy and love for the next generation. He is the "real deal" and a blessing not just to us, but to all who have ever come in contact with him.

Nashid Sharrief – Once a high school math teacher in Detroit, Nashid helped show us what's required to truly *empower*. Through his guidance, we now understand that the only way to achieve our mission is to not only empower teens but the parents and educators that support them as well.

Vince Coyner – All great products require collective effort, and an essential element is critical thinking. Vince has made us look at our conclusions differently. He has challenged every assumption in our work and driven our collective thinking forward immensely.

Wes Williams – Wes is an example of what we want for all youth. A successful businessman, he has given valuable time, energy, and resources to us unconditionally. There is no doubt the great successes in his life are a direct result of his powerful giving spirit.

Tim O'Rourke – Tim was one of the first to believe in our mission and commit himself to our cause. His support has given us great confidence in our work and motivated us to persevere through many trying times.

Pat Traynor – We were incredibly fortunate to meet Pat through one of our students. He is an incredible philanthropist and human being, and the support of someone of his reputation and character really validated our efforts. Pat's vision for North Dakota deeply inspired us and provided a launching point for our mission to impact millions.

Jorge Olmos – Jorge is our great blessing in Mexico. Passionate about teaching and empowering youth, he has helped us take the *7 Mindsets* to his country. Today, Mexico is one of our largest areas served outside of the United States, largely due to the wonderful work that Jorge is doing.

Lara Hodgson – An extraordinary woman, she is the great connector. Through her, we have created extraordinary relationships, met people we could only dream of meeting, and learned to create our dreams with and through others and their organizations.

Rand Cabus – The creative and artistic genius who gave life to many of our ideas, including book cover designs, logos, and countless items designed to empower and inspire youth to live their dreams.

Bernardo Flores – Perhaps the kindest young soul we have ever met. Bernardo provided us with critical input from a teenager's perspective. He also has inspired us in many ways and given us great confidence in our future, a future in the hands of extraordinary young men and women such as him.

Lourdes Mola – Thanks to Lourdes, we achieved extraordinary success with our flagship event, The Ultimate Life Summit, at Disney World. The experiment went on to become an incredible realization of our youth empowerment mission.

George Moore – Among the most extraordinary young people we have ever met, he has inspired us to take our message to Europe. Each day he drives us to do better, reach more youth, and maximize the positive impact we are having.

Stephanie Johnston – An incredible young woman from North Dakota, Stephanie has taught us how to bring our methodology into a community and work with all interested parties in creating a sustainable, positive impact at a local level.

Chris Koke – The creative spirit of our organization, Chris helped drive us to think differently; he consistently embodies many of the greatest aspects of our work. He is a man who has learned how to enjoy the moment and teaches us this lesson each and every day.

Adam Stern – A true hero to us, Adam was with us from day one. He persevered through many frustrations and stood by us through and through. He has been instrumental in so many aspects of our success, and we thank him for the gift of his time and positive energy.

Leslie Williams – Among our first supporters, she committed to our mission enthusiastically. She has brought us such joy and warm-heartedness. Since day one, she has embodied our mission and commitment to young people.

Ruth Baez – A wonderfully loving woman, she helped build our mission in the Dominican Republic and Latin America. Only through her could we have gotten mothers to believe in who we are. Never without a smile, she embodies everything we want to be.

Jorge Posada – One of our great heroes, Jorge is truly one of the ultra successful. In a life measured by joy in each moment, he is perhaps the most successful person we know. It is a gift to know him and a blessing to be part of his life.

Duane Moyer – An essential person at a critical time! Someone with the confidence to push the world around and the courage to accept feedback to help us all become better. Thank you, Duane, for being the catalyst.

David Craig – David joined our team in 2009 after supporting our work for years. One of our greatest assets, he helped us create sustainability in our mission, developing a business that will empower youth for many years to come. David is a great friend, and we look forward to our continued journey together.

Alice Ormiston – Often the unsung hero, Alice was closely involved for many years in everything we do. She has been instrumental in all of our successes and in every aspect of our business and foundation. She is a trusted advisor and provides the essential support that allows us to function at our best.

April Farlow – April is one of our great teachers. She has taught us how to be better and challenged us to get more from ourselves than we ever realized possible. We look forward to helping each other live our dreams together.

Tracey Smith – Tracey has an uncanny ability to define and execute a vision for a school. A truly inspiring leader, she is one of the best leaders we have come across. She's on the front lines, fighting the good fight and impacting the lives of young people every day.

Mimi Gamel – We are forever indebted to Mimi, the first educator crazy enough to give us a chance. Through the pilot at her school and her related research, she helped demonstrate how our concepts could positively impact academics, behavior, resilience and grit.

Mahmoud Dahy – Our prayers answered! Mahmoud Dahy was the much-needed technological genius we crossed paths with in 2012. He has single-handedly stabilized our products and placed us on the cutting edge of social and emotional learning solutions.

Michelle Weber – Who would have thought Fargo, North Dakota, would have been the genesis of our school programs? Only through the vision and efforts of Michelle Weber, an extraordinary principal and leader, were we able to validate our ability to implement *7 Mindsets* education in schools on a large scale.

Chelsea Buchanan – When our paths crossed in 2013, we were only working with middle and high school students. Chelsea had the first vision of the *7 Mindsets* in elementary schools and was integral in creating the elementary program at the core of some of our greatest successes.

Jadd Shickler – The best ideas cannot have an impact if no one hears about them. Jadd's proliferation, precision and attention to detail have allowed us to find our voice in sharing our story. His efforts have made it a certainty that the potential of the *7 Mindsets* will be fulfilled.

Ultimate Life Summit Students – All of our early development efforts center on the Ultimate Life Summit we conduct each year. We would like to thank each and every one of the students who have attended. You are the reason we do what we do. The future is bright because it is now in your hands.

Appendix A: People Interviewed and Studied

We researched and interviewed more than 400 individuals. Due to limited space, we are listing about 100 here. The complete list can be found at www.7Mindsets.com.

John Adams, Founding Father of the United States

*Mark Albion, Author, *Making A Life, Making A Living*

*Wally Amos, Founder, Famous Amos Cookies

Maya Angelou, Author and Poet

Aristotle, Greek Philosopher

Arthur Ashe, Champion Tennis Player

Mary Kay Ashe, Founder, Mary Kay Cosmetics

Marcus Aurelius, Roman Emperor and Philosopher

*Sir Richard Branson, Billionaire, Founder, The Virgin Group

*Les Brown, Motivational Speaker and Author, *Live Your Dreams*

*Marcus Buckingham, Author, *Now Discover Your Strengths*

Warren Buffet, Billionaire Investor and Author

*Jack Canfield, Co-Author, *Chicken Soup for the Soul*

Andrew Carnegie, American Industrialist and Businessman

Dr. Ben Carson, Neurosurgeon

Deepak Chopra, Author

Winston Churchill, WWII-era British Prime Minister

*Ben Cohen & Jerry Greenfield, Founders, Ben & Jerry's Ice Cream

*Jim Collins, Author, *Good to Great*

Confucius, Ancient Chinese Social Philosopher

Steven Covey, Author, *The 7 Habits of Highly Effective People*

Leonardo da Vinci, Renaissance Artist, Architect, Scientist, and Engineer

Henry David Thoreau, Famous American Author and Philosopher

*Fred DeLuca, Founder, SUBWAY®

Walt Disney, Founder, Walt Disney Company

*Wayne Dyer, Author

Amelia Earhart, First Woman to Fly Across the Atlantic

Thomas Edison, Industrialist and Inventor

Albert Einstein, Scientist

Ralph Waldo Emerson, Author and Philosopher

Appendix A: People Interviewed and Studied

Debbie Fields, Founder: Mrs. Fields Cookies

Anne Frank, Author and Victim of Holocaust

Viktor Frankl, Psychologist, Author, and Holocaust Survivor

Benjamin Franklin, American Founding Father, Inventor, and Author

Mahatma Gandhi, Political and Ideological Leader

Bill Gates, Co-Founder, Microsoft

*Michael Gerber, Author, *The E-Myth*

Khalil Gibran, Artist, Author and Poet

Jane Goodall, Internationally Acclaimed Primate Researcher

Alexander Graham Bell, Inventor of the Telephone

*Earl Graves, Founder, Black Enterprise Magazine

Bethany Hamilton, Teenage Surfer and Shark Attack Survivor

*Mark Victor Hansen, Co-Author, *Chicken Soup for the Soul*

Carlos Slim Helo, One of the Wealthiest Men in the World, Mexico

Napoleon Hill, Author, *Think and Grow Rich*

Patrick Henry Hughes, Inspirational Musician

Paul Hewson (Bono), Singer, U2, Humanitarian

*Wayne Huizenga, Entrepreneur, Owner, Miami Dolphins

Thomas Jefferson, Founding Father and 3rd President of the United States

Steve Jobs, Co-Founder, Apple Computers

Michael Jordan, Basketball Player

Helen Keller, Author and Political Activist

*Dennis Kimbro, Author, *What Makes the Great Great*

*Robert Kiyosaki, Entrepreneur, Author, *Rich Dad, Poor Dad*

Guy Laliberte, Founder, Cirque du Soleil

Dalai Lama, Spiritual Leader

Abraham Lincoln, 16th President of the United States

Martin Luther King, Jr., Civil Rights Leader

Nelson Mandela, President of South Africa

John Maxwell, Author and Leadership Coach

Michelangelo, Renaissance Artist, Architect, Poet, and Engineer

J. P. Morgan, Industrialist

Isaac Newton, Physicist

Earl Nightingale, Motivational Speaker

Norman Vincent Peale, Author

Pablo Picasso, Artist

*Daniel Pink, Author, *A Whole New Mind*

Plato, Philosopher

Bob Proctor, Author, Speaker and Life Coach

*Scott Rigsby, Ironman Triathlete

Shakira Mebarak Ripoll, Colombian Musician, Philanthropist

Appendix A: People Interviewed and Studied

Tony Robbins, Author, Speaker, and Life Coach

John Rockefeller, American Industrialist

*Anita Roddick, Founder, The Body Shop

Eleanor Roosevelt, Inspirational First Lady of the United States

William Rosenberg, Founder, Dunkin' Donuts

Joane (J.K.) Rowling, Author of Harry Potter Series

Wilma Rudolph, Olympic Gold Medalist

Rumi, Poet and Theologian

William Shakespeare, Renaissance Actor and Author

Mimi Silbert, Founder, Delancey Street Foundation

Will Smith, Actor

W. Clement Stone, Billionaire Businessman and Author

Mother Teresa, Philanthropist

*Dave Thomas, Founder, Wendy's

Eckhart Tolle, Author and Life Coach

*Brian Tracy, Author and Life Coach

Donald Trump, Businessman and Author

Ted Turner, Businessman and Author

Desmond Tutu, Political Activist

Mark Twain, Author and Speaker

Lao Tzu, Social Philosopher

Voltaire, Enlightenment Philosopher and Author

Nick Vujicic, Motivational Speaker

*Denis Waitley, Author and Life Coach

George Washington Carver, Scientist, Inventor and Educator

Jerry Weintraub, Hollywood Producer

Oprah Winfrey, Billionaire Talk Show Host

John Wooden, College Basketball Coach

Zhang Xin, Self-Made Female Billionaire, China

*Zig Ziglar, Author and Speaker

* These individuals were personally interviewed by our team.

Appendix B: Reference Books

Wally Amos, *The Power in You* (New York: Dutton Adult)

Andy Andrews, *The Butterfly Effect: How Your Life Matters* (Illinois: Simple Truths, LLC)

Andy Andrews *Mastering the Seven Decisions That Determine Personal Success* (Tennessee: Thomas Nelson Publishers)

Janet Bray Attwood and Chris Attwood, *The Passion Test: The Effortless Path to Discovering Your Destiny* (Iowa: 1st World Publishing)

Doug Bench, *Revolutionize Your Brain* (Florida: Doug Bench Enterprises)

Richard Branson, *Business Stripped Bare: Adventures of a Global Entrepreneur* (London: Penguin Books, Ltd.)

Richard Brodie, *Virus of the Mind: The New Science of the Meme* (California: Hay House)

Brendon Bruchard, *Life's Golden Ticket: An Inspirational Novel* (New York: HarperCollins)

Marcus Buckingham and Donald O. Clifton, *Now Discover Your Strengths* (New York: Simon & Schuster)

Bob Burg and John David Mann, *The Go-Giver: A Little Story About a Powerful Business Idea* (London: Penguin Books, Ltd.)

Jack Canfield and Kent Healy, *The Success Principles for Teens: How to Get From Where You Are to Where You Want to Be* (Florida: Health Communications, Inc.)

Jack Canfield and Janet Switzer, *The Success Principles: How to Get from Where You Are to Where You Want to Be* (New York, HarperCollins Publishers)

Jack Canfield and Mark Victor Hansen, *The Aladdin Factor* (New York: Berkley Publishing)

Dale Carnegie, *How to Win Friends and Influence People* (New York: Simon & Schuster)

Deepak Chopra, *The Seven Spiritual Laws of Success: A Pocketbook Guide to Fulfilling Your Dreams (One Hour Wisdom)* (California: Amber-Allen Publishing and New World Library)

Carol Christen and Richard N. Bolles, *What Color Is Your Parachute for Teens: Discovering Yourself, Defining Your Future* (California: Berkeley Press)

Bill Clinton, *Giving: How Each of Us Can Change the World* (Canada: Random House)

Paulo Coelho, *The Alchemist* (New York: HarperCollins)

Jim Collins, *Good to Great: Why Some Companies Make the Leap ... and Others Don't* (New York: HarperCollins)

Geoff Colvin, *Talent Is Overrated: What Really Separates World-Class Performers from Everybody Else* (New York: Penguin Group)

Stephen Covey, *The 7 Habits of Highly Effective People* (New York: Free Press)

Fred DeLuca and John P. Hays, *Start Small, Finish Big: 15 Key Lessons to Start—and Run—Your Own Business* (New York: Warner Business Books)

Dr. John Demartini, *The Gratitude Effect: The Inner Power Series* (TruMedia Group)

Carol Dweck, *Mindset: The New Psychology of Success* (New York: Ballentine)

Hale Dwoskin and Jack Canfield, *The Sedona Method: Your Key to Lasting Happiness, Success, Peace and Emotional Well-Being* (Arizona: Sedona Press)

Dr. Wayne Dyer, *Excuses Begone! How to Change Lifelong, Self-Defeating Thinking Habits* (California: Hayhouse)

Dr. Wayne Dyer, *The Power of Intention* (California: Hay House)

Ralph Waldo Emerson, *Self-Reliance: The Wisdom of Ralph Waldo Emerson as Inspiration of Daily Living* (New York: Bell Tower)

Mark Forstater, *The Spiritual Teaching of Marcus Aurelius* (New York: HarperCollins)

Marshall Frady, *Martin Luther King, Jr.: A Life* (New York: Viking Penguin)

Victor Frankl, *Man's Search for Meaning* (Massachusetts: Beacon Press)

Neal Gabler, *Walt Disney: The Triumph of American Imagination* (New York: Alfred Knopf)

Howard Gardner, *Frames of Mind: The Theory of Multiple Intelligences* (Pennsylvania: Perseus Books)

Michael J. Gelb, *How to Think Like Leonardo da Vinci* (New York: Dell Publishing)

Malcolm Gladwell, *Outliers: The Story of Success* (New York: Little, Brown and Company)

Shakti Gawain, *Creative Visualization: Use the Power of Imagination to Create What You Want in Your Life* (California, Nataraj Publishing)

Shakti Gawain, Marianne Williamson, and Mother Teresa, *For the Love of God* (California: Nataraj Publishing Company)

Mark Victor Hansen, *The Richest Kids in America: How They Earn It, How They Spend It, How You Can Too* (California: Hansen House)

Keith Harrell, *Attitude Is Everything, Rev Ed: 10 Life-Changing Steps to Turning Attitude into Action* (New York: HarperCollins)

Daren Hardy, *The Compound Effect: Multiplying Your Success, One Simple Step at a Time* (Texas: Success Books)

Dr. David R. Hawkins, *Power vs. Force: The Hidden Determinant of Human Behavior* (California: Hayhouse)

Tony Hsieh, *Delivering Happiness: A Path to Profits, Passion, and Purpose* (New York: Business Plus)

Napoleon Hill, *Think and Grow Rich* (New York: Plume)

Napoleon Hill and W. Clement Stone, *Success through a Positive Mental Attitude* (New York: Simon & Schuster)

Walter Isaacson, *Albert Einstein: His Life and Universe* (New York: Simon and Shuster)

Susan Jeffers Ph.D., *Feel the Fear ... and Do It Anyway* (New York: Ballentine)

Paul Johnson, *Churchill* (New York: Viking)

Willie Jolley, *It Only Takes a Minute to Change Your Life* (New York: St. Martin's Press)

Michael Jordan and Mark Vancil, *I Can't Accept Not Trying: Michael Jordan on the Pursuit of Excellence* (California: Harper)

Helen Keller, *The Story of My Life* (New York: Doubleday)

Dennis Kimbro, *Think and Grow Rich: A Black Choice* (New York: Fawcett Books)

Dennis Kimbro, *What Makes the Great Great* (New York: Main Street Books)

Martin Luther King, Jr., *The Autobiography of Martin Luther King, Jr., Ed. Clayborne Carson* (New York: Warner Books, Inc.)

Charles G. Koch, *The Science of Success: How Market-Based Management Built the World's Largest Private Company* (New Jersey: John Wiley & Sons)

Jennifer Kushell, *Secrets of the Young and Successful* (Princeton

Review)

Robert Kiyosaki, *Rich Dad Poor Dad: What the Rich Teach Their Kids About Money That the Poor and Middle Class Do Not!* (TechPress)

H.H. Dalai Lama, *The Art of Happiness* (New York: Riverhead Books)

Ellen J. Langer, *Mindfulness* (Pennsylvania: Perseus Books Group)

Bruce H. Lipton, Ph.D., *The Biology of Belief: Unleashing the Power of Consciousness, Matter, and Miracles* (California: Hay House)

Nelson Mandela, *Long Walk to Freedom: The Autobiography of Nelson Mandela* (New York: Back Bay Books)

John Maxwell, *Talent Is Never Enough: Discover the Choices that Will Take You Beyond Your Talent* (Tennessee: Thomas Nelson)

John Maxwell, *The 21 Irrefutable Laws of Leadership* (Tennessee: Thomas Nelson)

George McGovern, *Abraham Lincoln* (New York: Times Books)

Jay McGraw, *Life Strategies for Teens* (New York: Fireside)

Dr. Phil McGraw, *Life Strategies: Doing What Works, Doing What Matters* (New York: Hyperion)

James M. McPherson, *Abraham Lincoln and the 2nd American Revolution* (New York: Oxford University Press)

Dan Millman, *The Way of the Peaceful Warrior: A Book That Changes Lives* (Navoto, California, H.J. Kramer)

Stephen Mitchell, *The Tao Te Ching: A New English Version* (New York: HarperCollins)

Greg Mortenson, *Three Cups of Tea* (New York: Penguin Books)

Joseph Murphy, *The Power of Your Subconscious Mind* (New York: Bantam)

Lisa Nichols, *No Matter What! 9 Steps to Living the Life You Love* (New York: Hachette Book Group)

Dr. Norman Vincent Peale, *The Power of Positive Thinking* (New York: Fireside)

M. Scott Peck, M.D., *The Road Less Traveled: A New Psychology of Love, Traditional Values and Spiritual Growth* (New York: Touchstone)

Daniel Pink, *Drive: The Surprising Truth About What Motivates Us* (New York: Riverhead Books)

Daniel Pink, *A Whole New Mind: Why Right-Brainers Will Rule the Future* (New York: Berkley Publishing)

Steven Pinker, *The Stuff of Thought: Language as a Window into Human Nature* (New York: Penguin Publishing)

James Redfield, *The Celestine Prophecy* (New York: Warner Books)

Scott Rigsby, *Unthinkable* (Illinois: Tyndale House)

Alexandra Robbins and Ab Wilner, *Quarterlife Crisis: The Unique Challenges of Life in Your Twenties* (New York: Jeremy P. Tarcher/Putnam)

Anthony Robbins, *Awaken the Giant Within: How to Take Immediate Control of Your Mental, Emotional, Physical and Financial Destiny!* (New York: Free Press)

Anthony Robbins, *Unlimited Power: The New Science of Personal Achievement* (New York: Free Press)

Ken Robinson, Ph.D., *The Element: How Finding Your Passion Changes Everything* (New York: Penguin Publishing)

Jim Rohn, *Three Keys to Greatness for Teenagers* (audible edition: Made for Success, Inc.)

Jim Rohn, *The Art of Exceptional Living* (Illinois: Nightingale-Conant)

Miguel Ruiz, *The Four Agreements: A Practical Guide to Personal Freedom* (California: Amber-Allen Publishing, Inc.)

SQuire Rushnell, *When GOD Winks: How the Power of Coincidence Guides Your Life* (New York: Atria Books)

Martin E.P. Seligman, *Authentic Happiness: Using the New Positive*

Psychology to Realize Your Potential for Deep Fulfillment (Boston: Nicholas Brealey)

Martin E.P. Seligman, Ph.D., *Learned Optimism: How to Change Your Mind and Your Life* (New York: Simon & Schuster)

Marci Shimoff, *Happy for No Reason: 7 Steps to Being Happy from the Inside Out* (New York: Free Press)

Florence Scovel Shinn, *The Game of Life and How to Play It*, (Tribeca Books)

Sam Smith, *The Jordan Rules* (New York: Pocket Books)

Mother Teresa and Brian Kolodiejchuk, *Come Be My Light* (New York: Random House)

Eckhart Tolle, *The Power of Now* (Canada: Namaste Publishing)

Eckhart Tolle, *A New Earth* (New York: Penguin Publishing)

W. Clement Stone and Michael Ritt, *Believe and Achieve: W. Clement Stone's 17 Principles of Success* (Pennsylvania: Executive Books)

Lao Tzu and Brian Brown Walker, *The Tao Te Ching Lao Tzu* (New York: St. Martin's Press)

Brian Tracy, *Maximum Achievement: Strategies and Skills that Will Unlock Your Hidden Power to Succeed* (New York: Fireside)

Christiane Turner, *Quantum NLP: From Personal to Global Transformation* (New York: Gilden Media)

Neale Donald Walsch, *Conversations with God* (New York: Penguin Publishing)

Rick Warren, *The Purpose Driven Life: What on Earth Am I Here For?* (Michigan: Zondervan)

Liz Wiseman and Greg McKeown, *Multipliers: How the Best Leaders Make Everyone Smarter* (New York: HarperCollins)

Steve Young, *Great Failures of the Extremely Successful: Mistake, Adversity, Failure and Other Stepping Stones to Success* (California: Tallfellow Press)

Muhammad Yunus, *Banker to the Poor: Micro-Lending and the Battle Against Poverty* (New York: Public Affairs)

More Praise for
The 7 Mindsets to Live Your Ultimate Life:

"The *7 Mindsets* represent a phenomenal construction that changed my perception and elevated my potential to achieve my goals in a manner that I was never exposed to before. Their power lies in altering the negative evaluation of one's personal attributes into progressive outlooks that fundamentally help in self-improvement and, subsequently, in communal development. I believe that if the *7 Mindsets* were introduced to the youth here in the United Arab Emirates, the outcome would be truly rewarding."

Fatma Alshowab
Graduate Student, United Arab Emirates

"An extreme amplification of happiness, success, motivation and service came to my life after being exposed to the *7 Mindsets*. These mindsets are so clear and efficient that making them a lifestyle is extremely easy and helpful."

Karen Carvajalino Martinez
Student, Colombia

"The *7 Mindsets* have opened my mind and thousands of doors that will lead to success in my life. They have opened my eyes and helped me know that I will reach my fullest potential. I wish so much that more students from the Dominican Republic could share my experience."

Carla Rodriguez Dajer
Student, Dominican Republic

157

"Not just a set of ideas, but a way of living. The *7 Mindsets* teach you how to live a happier and more successful life. They've taught me that happiness is not the destination, it's the journey."

George Moore
Student, London, England

"The *7 Mindsets* are based on principles that are critical to helping unlock mental barriers that keep the majority of people from experiencing fulfilled, successful lives. Since my exposure to the *7 Mindsets*, I have used them personally to inspire new ideas and solidify my attitude to succeed professionally. I also use them to inspire and encourage youth. Through great stories and the scientific research to back up the results, the *7 Mindsets* will awaken the hope to achieve your personal definition of success!"

Lazarus Bruner, Jr.
Educator/Entrepreneur

"The *7 Mindsets* showed me a different way to see and experience life, especially a different way to treat people and live my passion."

Stephanie Carvajalino Martinez
Student, Colombia

"I have always strived to reach my full potential, but it wasn't until I dug deep into the *7 Mindsets* that I realized my potential is unlimited! I now truly believe everything is possible when one holds a positive mindset. I've been inspired to dream bigger than ever before, and to take action to achieve my biggest dreams."

Stephanie Johnston
Student, Fargo, North Dakota

"I have seen the radical and positive change among youth while living the *7 Mindsets*. Learning them is truly a life-changing experience. They are a practical guide to positive personal challenges for all of us with a global vision, and to positive change."

Jorge Olmos
Educator, Mexico City, Mexico